Plague-Making and the AIDS Epidemic

Plague-Making and the AIDS Epidemic: A Story of Discrimination

Gina M. Bright

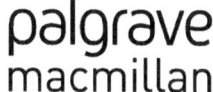
palgrave
macmillan

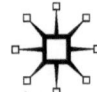
First published in 2012 by
PALGRAVE MACMILLAN®
in the United States—a division of St. Martin's Press LLC,
175 Fifth Avenue, New York, NY 10010.

Where this book is distributed in the UK, Europe and the rest of the World,
this is by Palgrave Macmillan, a division of Macmillan Publishers Limited,
registered in England, company number 785998, of Houndmills,
Basingstoke, Hampshire RG21 6XS.

Palgrave Macmillan is the global academic imprint of the above
companies and has companies and representatives throughout the world.

Palgrave® and Macmillan® are registered trademarks in the United
States, the United Kingdom, Europe and other countries.

ISBN: 978–0–230–34071–8

Library of Congress Cataloging-in-Publication Data

Bright, Gina M., 1965–
    Plague-making and the AIDS epidemic : a story of discrimination/
Gina M. Bright.
        p.   ;   cm.
    Includes bibliographical references.
    ISBN 978–0–230–34071–8 (alk. paper)
    I. Title. [DNLM: 1. HIV Infections—psychology—Europe.
2. HIV Infections—psychology—United States. 3. Prejudice—
Europe. 4. Prejudice—United States. 5. HIV Infections—
history—Europe. 6. HIV Infections—history—United States.
7. Plague—history—Europe. 8. Plague—history—United States.
9. Plague—psychology—Europe. 10. Plague—psychology—
United States.   WC 503.7]
    LC classification not assigned
    614.5/99392–dc23   2011032893

A catalogue record of the book is available from the British Library.

Design by Integra Software Services

First edition: February 2012

For Cisco and all the others: This is your story.

Contents

Acknowledgments

I am deeply indebted to a few people in the writing of this book. My husband, Mike, was the first and only reader of the book for years. I will spend the rest of my life thanking him for his intellectual and emotional support, his editorial suggestions, and his love, especially during the darker moments. My dog, Wat, provided lap support through several chapters. My sister, Wendy, and her husband, Joe, always lent a supportive ear and good times for relief. As usual, my parents provided an unending well of emotional support. Dr. Patricia Ingham continues to influence my intellectual and political thought years after she kindly served as my teacher, doctoral studies director, and friend. Every one of the hundreds of people with AIDS I have cared for inspired me to return to my writing table every day, year after year until the book was completed. It is a testimony to their struggles, losses, and triumphs over the past three decades.

PART I

Introduction

CHAPTER 1

Why I Wrote This Book

The history of acquired immune deficiency syndrome (AIDS) is a history of discrimination. The unfortunate labeling of AIDS as a plague when the epidemic emerged in the early 1980s has engendered much of the discrimination experienced by people who have lived, and are living, with the syndrome or the human immunodeficiency virus (HIV).

I was introduced to AIDS in the summer of 1982, on the verge of entering my senior year of high school. One afternoon that summer I happened to see a guest on the *Phil Donahue* show loudly claim that a mysterious new disease was ravaging the male homosexual community in New York City. This man turned out to be Larry Kramer, one of the cofounders of *Gay Men's Health Crisis*—a foundation created in 1981 by and for gay men that provides legal, emotional, and medical support for people with AIDS—and later one of the most important and incendiary AIDS activists. He was calling for some sort of attention, *any* attention, to be given to this new disease. As I was 17 years old and growing up in a suburban area of eastern Pennsylvania, I tried to understand why the disease, which apparently shut down the immune system and resulted in a rare form of cancer and pneumonia, was primarily infecting gay men. I grew angry as I listened to Kramer explain that local health authorities and the government were ignoring his community. "How could anyone ignore such a frightening new disease that seemed to be affecting so many people?" I thought. When my mother arrived home from work, I was in a state of concern bordering on panic. She responded with her perennial optimism, the type of response I have actually grown to admire over subsequent years if for the only reason that it infuses rationality into my oftentimes cynical worldview: "Well, Gina, don't exaggerate. It doesn't sound *that* bad since only a few people have the disease now. Someone will find a cure."

All of us who have been affected by AIDS—whether we live with the disease; are the mother, father, sister, brother, spouse, lover, or friend of someone who has it or did have it; or have cared for people with AIDS—certainly now, three decades after its appearance, wish that my mother's optimistic response had become a reality. But it did not. Nonetheless, when I first heard about this new disease in 1982, only a few hundred people had contracted it in the United States and more than 100 people had died from it; by the mid-1980s, the number of people living with AIDS and those who died from it remained well under 50,000.[1] I highlight this not to diminish, by any means, anyone who has been diagnosed with AIDS or who has died from it, but only to introduce the notion that in spite of a relatively small number of people contracting AIDS in mid-1980s America, this disease was being constructed as a plague, even *the* plague.

The first reported cases of what a few years later would be known as AIDS appeared in the June 5 and July 3, 1981, editions of the *Morbidity and Mortality Weekly Report,* the medical field's necrologue or weekly report on existing and emerging diseases and deaths. In June 1981, five young homosexual men were reported to have *Pneumocystis carinii* pneumonia (PCP), a rare form of pneumonia often seen in patients who have compromised immune systems from chemotherapy. And in the July report, 26 homosexual men were reported to have a rare form of cancer, Kaposi's sarcoma, usually seen in its classic and nonaggressive form in older men of Mediterranean descent.[2]

By mid-1983, however, with less than one thousand people infected with AIDS and less than four hundred people dead from the disease, the gay community and some politically conservative judges of nontraditional sexual behaviors were calling AIDS the "gay plague."[3] It is quite understandable that the gay community initially would choose the word "plague" for this new disease. In mid-1983, people infected with AIDS were primarily concentrated in large urban areas such as New York City, Los Angeles, and San Francisco, and these gay communities were witnessing death on a daily basis. So it is no surprise that "plague" aptly described the horrors they were experiencing. After all, the term has been used to describe many deadly diseases throughout the history of Western civilization. In particular, the bubonic plague swept across Europe, Western Asia, the Middle East, and Africa in the mid-fourteenth century, killing what is most recently believed to be at least 62 percent of the European population alone.[4] Other diseases such as yellow fever, measles, small pox, and even polio have been labeled "plagues" because they killed or affected large numbers of people in relatively short periods of time. Small pox alone killed more than 300 million people in the twentieth century before it was eradicated in the late 1970s. Even the 1918 influenza epidemic has been categorized more recently as a "plague." The H5N1 influenza strain is thought to have killed anywhere from 20 to approximately 100 million people across the world from 1918 to 1919.[5]

Chances are that if you were not living in a major city or did not have ties with the gay community in 1983, you did not know anyone living with or dying from AIDS—like I did not, yet. References to AIDS as the "gay plague" by nonmembers of an urban or gay community did not stem from a familiarity with people suffering with this disease, but from something far more sinister: an intolerant belief system.

The executive vice president of the Moral Majority in Lynchburg, Virginia, said in June 1983 that the government needs to allot more funds to "protect" the general public from the "gay plague."[6] The Moral Majority was a highly conservative Christian fundamentalist political organization created in 1979 by Jerry Falwell for the sole purpose of gaining political votes on issues that would maintain inequality for women and homosexuals. Its executive vice president believed that prohibiting gay men from donating blood would cocoon all blood recipients from the disease, whereas money spent only on medical research would allow "these diseased homosexuals to go back to their perverted practices without any standards of accountability."[7] Identifying and controlling the sexual practices of gay men was the main platform of this "moral" man's epidemiologic program. The label of "plague" for AIDS here is based neither on the actual contagiousness of the disease—after all, the general public can be protected if gay men simply do not donate blood—nor on the number of people who have been infected (by mid-1983 only 1,450 cases were reported).[8] The sexual practices of non-heterosexual men inspired the usage of this term.

Even more appalling was a statement made by a New Orleans medical doctor around the same time. In a conversation with a colleague, this doctor pondered whether or not AIDS was "God's punishment," saying that "if it is, it is not harsh enough."[9] Statements like this, another testimony to intolerant beliefs and value judgments about the gay community, echo the views of chroniclers in fourteenth-century Europe who wrote about bubonic plague when it swept that continent. A Russian chronicle of the bubonic plague in the spring of 1352 described the inhabitants of Pskov petitioning the archbishop to visit and bless their town because they "were without any means of averting this punishment from God."[10] Most fourteenth-century writers viewed the plague as God's punishment for committed sins. What constituted a sin in the fourteenth century was not so different from now, and the New Orleans doctor's notion that God punishes a certain segment of the population for unorthodox behavior with diseases like AIDS points to a plague mentality reminiscent of these medieval attitudes. Labeling AIDS a "plague," especially a gay one, means a great deal more than benignly describing an infectious disease that quickly kills a large number of people.

In 1985, I cared for my first AIDS patient when I was in my last year of nursing school in eastern Pennsylvania and working extra shifts on the weekend in the hospital where I was training. One Saturday evening, I reported for duty on the oncology ward, where I always met people infected with HIV and still do today. The assignments for that evening were distributed and I quickly noticed that my one patient did not have the typical cancer diagnosis. There was red ink on the Kardex—the nursing profession's now obsolete recipe card for the care to be delivered to each patient every shift. I read the red phrases: "infected with HIV", "contact" isolation, and "respiratory" isolation. I must admit I was a little scared as I read these precautions, while at the same time filled with the anticipation of caring for someone with this relatively new illness that we still did not know that much about.

What we did know in 1985 was that AIDS was caused by a virus that finally, after much politicized scientific debate between American and French researchers, was named human immunodeficiency virus. We knew this virus was not readily, if at all, transmissible by casual contact (such as touching, hugging, and even kissing), although there was always talk about the virus being spread by the saliva of those infected. So I entered this young man's room confused by all of the infection control warnings on his door and by the dictates of the Kardex to wear a mask, gown, and gloves. Although he was being ruled out for tuberculosis, a highly infectious respiratory illness that made its unfortunate comeback in people with weakened immune systems, I understood the need for a mask but not for the gown and gloves if bodily fluids were not encountered. Tuberculosis had practically been eradicated in the Unites States, along with sanatoriums that housed the disease's victims, by the 1950s when effective antibiotic treatments were discovered. I wore the gloves anyway—at least in the beginning of my shift—and entered the room to introduce myself and perform my initial assessment of the patient.

I met a nice young gentleman who was much too thin and had been living in New York City. He had suddenly fallen ill with rapid weight loss, diarrhea, cough, and fever, and consequently returned home to Pennsylvania. He had a sister by his bedside but his parents were noticeably absent. Throughout my shift, this man had an increasingly difficult time breathing, and it was quickly becoming obvious that he needed respiratory support in the intensive care unit downstairs. However, before that transfer occurred later in the evening, I grew to understand that he was scared and had faced a great deal of discrimination from both his parents and the hospital staff. His parents were absent *because* of his disease. The dietary department left his dinner trays outside of his room on the floor. Some nurses and doctors did not even want to enter his room; some simply did not.[11] Not everyone in the medical field then, and even today, has witnessed this discrimination because of limited exposure to this patient population. But those of us who cared for patients with AIDS in the 1980s and subsequent decades have witnessed this trajectory of severe to more mild forms of neglect in their care.

After all, by 1985 AIDS was no longer the "gay plague"; it was being touted as "the new plague."[12] It seemed to be everywhere. Now children had AIDS and were not being allowed to attend school in several states. A famous actor had been infected with the disease. Even though the media forced Rock Hudson's sexual orientation onto the grand stage, AIDS was infecting people other than homosexuals, and the common reaction to the word "AIDS" was panic bordering on hysteria.

By the time I transferred this young man to the intensive care unit, I removed my gloves to hold his hand and assure him that he would be just fine. Of course at the time—actually until the mid-1990s with the advent of several new antiretroviral drugs that would keep this virus's power at bay—this was false assurance, but he needed it. More importantly, he needed someone behind all of that protective gear to make the smallest gesture of acceptance that he was simply a human being who *happened* to contract a horrible illness and not a human being who *deserved* this illness.

There were plenty of other health-care professionals in 1985 who touched people with AIDS without wearing gloves. Those of us who did actually believed what we read in the medical journals: The virus was not spread by casual contact. Those of us who did not were to some degree infected with the plague mentality that was enveloping the consciousness of America.

When the transport was completed, I said my first good-bye of many hundred more to AIDS patients. He and his sister thanked me for caring for him. I also think that they were deeply grateful that I held his hand without my gloves. I thank this patient for my first opportunity to care for someone suffering from AIDS. I thank him for introducing me to what it feels like to be treated like a plague carrier. And I thank him for always reminding me, to this day, that the simplest way to begin to overturn the plague mentality surrounding this disease is to extend a gloveless hand.

My particular focus in this book will be the AIDS epidemic in the United States, not only because I experienced firsthand the worst years of it here but also because American journalism, medical writings, film, literature, and other art forms created and perpetuated this epidemic as a plague. This is not to say that AIDS has not been treated as a plague in other countries, especially in Africa. But a close analysis of American reporting and art focusing on the epidemic reveals that the genesis of AIDS as a plague is closely bound to perceptions of and reactions to behaviors not readily accepted by mainstream society. Perhaps I forgot to mention that my first AIDS patient was a homosexual cross-dresser.

In order to understand how and why AIDS was *made* a plague, we will journey back to the centuries when other plagues, mainly bubonic, wreaked havoc on so many populations and imprinted the horrors of contagion, suffering, and death on the imaginations of history and literary writers. These supposedly bygone cultural reactions to plague reverberate in America with the entrance of AIDS into our society.

Viewing the AIDS epidemic as a plague actually has crippled our thoughts about and our feelings toward those people who have lived and are living with AIDS. My hope for the uninfected reader of this book is that if you ever meet someone with HIV or AIDS, your first reaction is not fear and blame but acceptance: acceptance that someone was unlucky enough to have contracted this virus and acceptance that it was not his or her fault. In these pages, I even encourage admiration for people living with a virus that constantly wages war on their immune systems, people who often fight to get out of bed and who try to fend off the uncomfortable nausea and oftentimes relentless diarrhea that can be among the unfortunate side-effects of the drugs that now keep them alive. These more rational responses to AIDS have in part been achieved in the United States as the days of meal trays left outside of patients' rooms, nurses and doctors refusing to or only reluctantly caring for these patients, and the infected children prohibited from attending school have become memories. But remnants of the dark ages of the epidemic still persist as the plague label rears its head in the discourse of politicians, journalists and other writers, and even medical experts. And the plague mentality still lurks in the conscience of many infected people who do not feel comfortable enough to openly discuss their viral status. My hope for the infected reader is that I manage to capture and expose the discrimination experienced by all of you who have been treated like plague carriers.

In 1989, I cared for a very talented dancer who was battling his second bout of PCP in an AIDS unit in New York City. His bed was situated in an old-style hospital wardroom with two beds on each side of the room facing each other. Certainly, these wards were not the ideal architectural space for four immuno-compromised patients as it exposed them to one another's opportunistic infections. This structural arrangement of beds was one testament to the medical community's neglect then of the best standard of care for AIDS patients.

I was working the night shift and this night was particularly intense: A patient in one room was experiencing respiratory failure and was ready to be placed on a ventilator to mechanically infuse his lungs with the oxygen his own body could not provide. In the dancer's four-bed room one patient was wasting away, weighing a mere 80 pounds and expelling what seemed to be endless liters of fecal matter. Another roommate was screaming and attempting to strike anyone who approached his bed as the virus infected his brain, turning everyone into an enemy. The dancer was standing in the middle of this room, shocked by the scene but composing himself emotionally and even attempting to help the less fortunate men there who had all been brought together by this disease. I was so thankful that the dancer, the muscles in his legs and arms still sculpted by his art, was healthy enough not to need my immediate care so I could focus on the more desperate needs of these other patients. He looked at me and asked, "Gina, are you getting all of this down?" He knew that I was studying English literature at the time, and I knew what he meant but I wanted to be sure: "What do you mean exactly?" "Are you writing all of this down, what we're going through? This is crazy." I responded, "I can't write it now, but I will one day." He replied, "Good, because we need you to tell our story."

I do not know whether the story in these pages is exactly what this patient had in mind. He certainly was aware of and experienced the discrimination that accompanied the diagnosis of AIDS in the 1980s. I remember that night and many more that were far worse and some that were a bit better. Mainly, I remember how much we—and I mean me and the other nurses with whom I was fortunate enough to work during all those years on that unit on those dark nights—cared for and fought for these patients. And I mean fought. We fought for their meal trays to be delivered directly to their rooms, for medical interns to visit them when they had high fevers, and for our own families' and friends' understanding of why we chose to take care of this patient population.

We fought a plague mentality. This book explores how this mentality erupted, persisted, and is responsible for the bulk of discrimination endured by persons with AIDS. Cisco, this is your story.

CHAPTER 2

What Is Plague?

Near the end of 1991, a nurse I worked with was quite distressed about the acuity of medical problems our patients with AIDS had endured over the past few weeks. We were caring for a man in his thirties housed in a private room with a B-cell lymphoma—a type of cancer of the white blood cells commonly affecting people with full-blown AIDS—actively eroding his right armpit from the inside out. We could smell his rotting flesh as we walked on to the unit at the far end of the hallway, and we were distraught by his intractable suffering. He had so much pain in spite of the intravenous Morphine infusion he received, and no matter how much pain medication the doctors ordered for his comfort, he did not achieve solace. At this time, there were a few other patients on the unit who were slowly fading away from wasting syndrome—an end-stage condition of AIDS involving uncontrollable diarrhea and vomiting and extreme weight loss in spite of receiving nutritional and other medical support.

One evening, this nurse approached me at the nurses' station: "I swear, Gina," she said, "this couldn't be anything other than plague." I asked her what she meant. "There are so many young people contracting, and dying from, this disease," she replied. In 1991, 29,850 people in the United States died from AIDS.[1] Granted, we were working in a New York City hospital and cared for what seemed to be the bulk of this statistic, especially in the 25–44-year-old age group in which AIDS was the third leading cause of death at the time. But do 30,000 deaths from an illness in a country with—at the time—approximately 250 million people qualify it as a plague? All of us were certainly nothing but stunned by the number of people admitted to our unit with AIDS, and even more shocked by the suffering they endured during a time when AZT, those blue and white capsules administered every four hours around the clock, was the only antiretroviral option for halting the virus' replication.

My colleague's pronouncement that AIDS was a plague intrigued and confused me that night, especially since I was also studying fourteenth-century bubonic plague in my undergraduate history and English literature courses. Bubonic plague, like AIDS, stole so many lives after causing not dissimilar symptoms such as high fevers; night sweats; and large, painful swellings at lymph node sites. I vaguely felt that AIDS might be a plague because of the number of deaths we personally witnessed, the celerity of the disease's progression then, and the fact that those Kaposi's sarcoma (KS) lesions indelibly imprinted on so many patients bears a resemblance to the buboes produced by the so-called plague bacillus.

But something about labeling AIDS as a plague disturbed me greatly in 1991, probably because a good amount of written material focusing on AIDS throughout the 1980s and the early 1990s often evoked this label to describe the disease in ways that did not produce sympathy or even empathy for its victims. In general, newspaper and magazine article descriptions of AIDS as a plague tended to produce feelings of fear, even panic, and worst of all *blame*: a notion that these people simply deserved what they got.

Almost a decade later, while pursuing graduate degrees in English literature back in eastern Pennsylvania, I worked on weekends and during the summer in a variety of institutions. Although I no longer cared solely for AIDS patients then, I, however, continued to meet people with this disease in the institutions that I worked. Of course by 1999, people with the virus had more drug options that greatly altered the debilitating course of full-blown AIDS and even prevented conversion to AIDS, but discriminatory perceptions of AIDS persisted. In several institutions I noticed that typical responses to AIDS patients by medical staff were blame for certain behaviors and a fairly extreme fear of contagion. As I was working the evening shift in a rehabilitation hospital, I overheard some nurses discussing a patient in whispering tones: "He will not open up to anyone"; "I wonder how he got it." Nurses in more suburban areas, like this hospital, did not have substantial contact with AIDS patients and many were greatly influenced, as the rest of American society was, by the cascade of emotions that had been produced by the media's presentation of AIDS. So I asked these nurses to discuss this patient with me; of course, I suspected that he was at least HIV positive but his viral status was rather incidental to his primary orthopedic diagnosis, the reason for his admission to this hospital. The problem was that none of the nurses were able to connect with this patient, or form a trusting relationship, in order to help him with his postoperative recovery. These nurses did not know me very well as I was working through an agency and not as a permanent staff member, and I informed them of my AIDS background in New York. I subsequently asked if anyone had any physical contact with this patient such as helping him out of bed to the chair. They said that any contact had been conducted with gloves even when bodily secretions were not encountered. I suggested that he might be more receptive if gloves were not used while just holding his arms, which did not have any wounds, and perhaps if on occasion people just sat down next to him in the chair by his bed and struck up casual conversations like they did with HIV negative patients on the unit.

I am not really sure if my simple advice to attempt to close the gap between this patient and the nursing staff was received, especially since I was not assigned to this unit again for a few months, but before the evening concluded I could not resist meeting this patient. I shook his hand without gloves and engaged him in a general conversation about his surgery and eventual recovery. I had no doubt that with this approach by other nurses the patient would have "opened up" to the staff and his recovery program as he began to do with me.

Almost two decades after AIDS emerged in the United States, I admit I was rather amazed to discover health-care workers approaching AIDS patients as plague carriers: These nurses were afraid to touch this patient and were concerned with the manner in which he contracted the virus. Of course even if they had known that this patient was a recovering intravenous drug abuser, they might not have castigated him for that behavior, but the curiosity about the route of transmission in contracting the virus suggested that some sort of judgment would have ensued. I must admit that all of us who worked on the AIDS unit in New York City asked about the route of viral transmission as part of our routine assessments. Of course, in the 1980s the medical community was still establishing and solidifying all groups at risk for HIV infection. But I persisted in this line of inquiry long after risk groups were established, until an AIDS activist I met in a research position I held in 2004 highlighted the discriminatory nature of the question itself. Perhaps I did not escape the plague mentality surrounding AIDS.

What exactly is *plague*, and why is this word capable of producing less than rational reactions in those who encounter it? Attempting to define plague is the first step in understanding many of the perceptions of AIDS I have described thus far. However, articulating a clear definition is challenging because the word possesses several meanings that do not necessarily coalesce into a unified one, or at least coalesce into one that explains the potential hazards of employing this word.

Perhaps it is easier to begin by defining what plague is not: a specific disease. This assertion may alarm members of the medical community who may well retort: "But there is bubonic plague." In reality what has been traditionally labeled bubonic, pneumonic, and even septicemic plague by medical scientists is the disease caused by *Yersinia pestis*, a bacterium discovered in the nineteenth century, and now usually cured with antibiotics. Although medical professionals know that this disease is caused by this bacterium, the disease consistently retains the label "plague." Yersinia disease, like AIDS, has been enveloped in cultural clouds of religious, social, and even ethnic perspectives that have steered the persistent application of the *plague* label and produced its consequences.

A brief and selective genealogy of thought about plague in Western cultures, both written fiction and nonfiction, will generate a workable definition for this word, and further assist in understanding older views of plague that eventually, sometimes noticeably and sometimes subtly, influenced twentieth-century American views of AIDS.

An appropriate place to begin is with Homer's *The Iliad*, the first epic poem produced by ancient Greek society. The poem focuses on the final conflict of the famous, and not easily dated, Trojan War, which was fought for ten years between the Greeks and the Trojans because Paris, a Trojan, kidnapped the wife of Menelaus, the legendary Greek beauty, Helen. This poem was composed between the eighth and seventh centuries BCE and was available as a written text by the end of the sixth century BCE. *The Iliad* most notably begins with plague that affects the Greek general, Agamemnon, and his army who have been waiting in siege outside of the city of Troy for nine years. Agamemnon has angered Chryses, a Trojan man who happens to be a devoted priest of the god Apollo, by making this priest's daughter his mistress. Chryses, of course, wants his daughter returned to him but Agamemnon refuses his requests, and consequently several men and animals within the Greek army are assaulted with and killed by the burning arrows of Apollo.

The actual barrage of burning arrows is called a "plague" by Achilles, one of the most famous and powerful Greek soldiers.[2] He advises Agamemnon to turn the Greeks homeward in order to save their lives from this additional source of danger. Achilles' description of the deadly arrows as a plague captures the first definition of plague offered by the *Oxford English Dictionary*, the authoritative dictionary detailing the etymology of English words and tracing their usages over the past millennium: "a blow, a stroke, a wound."[3] Homer's poem may fall outside of the historical scope of the *OED*, but these burning arrows afflicting the Greek army certainly wield "a blow" as "the corpse fires burned everywhere."[4]

Plague acquires another meaning in the first 100 lines of Homer's poem and likewise echoed in the *OED*: a deserved divine punishment. Apollo, who was generally thought of by Greek society as the god of music and archery, was also the god of healing, light, and Truth. In *The Iliad* he specifically appears as the divine being who administers a punishment for the Greeks:

"He [Apollo] came as night comes down and knelt then/apart and opposite the ships and let go an arrow."[5]

The divine punishment in the form of burning arrows is not haphazardly bestowed upon the Greek army by Apollo; it is deserved because of Agamemnon's violation of a Trojan girl. Achilles suspects that this occurrence of *plague*, as he has called it, is not gratuitous. This was confirmed by Kalchas, a seer who resides within the Greek camp, who when asked to explain the reason for this deadly blow to the Greeks tells Achilles that this "shameful plague"[6] will not abate until Agamemnon returns Chryses' daughter. The plague is the visible signifier of the Greeks' disrespect of an innocent Trojan girl and it is well-deserved retribution for this behavior, according to this seer. The plague ceases when Agamemnon returns the girl to her father and the Greeks offer gifts to Apollo.

Divine causes of plague are frequently offered by different societies to explain the suffering caused by it, and in particular to provoke a change in the particular behavior that was perceived as the incitement for this divine punishment, as Homer shows us here. Human causes of plague are also proposed by different societies, and this poem suggests that the divine being might not have caused the plague without human influence. Chryses, after all, is one of Apollo's priests, and after his initial request to the Greeks to allow him to take his daughter home to Troy is denied, he prays to Apollo for their punishment: "let your arrows make the Danaans [Greeks] pay for my shed tears."[7] Chryses is a human source of plague but he remains unaffected by it as he does not endure the deadly sting of the burning arrows, and he is even vindicated by the plague when his daughter is returned to him by the suffering Greek army. Homer's poem may be unique in offering a human cause of plague who is not disparaged and assigned blame by the social group experiencing the punishment. In other earlier and later Western texts, proposed human sources of plague are usually in the position of the enemy or at least the marginalized.

An artist in any given society does not live in a vacuum; rather, he or she experiences those ideas, values, and mores that are expressed, to varying degrees, in the art produced. For the ancient Greek society in which Homer lived, plague was not a disease but a physical assault, with both a divine and human cause, to be endured by a group of people until certain behaviors were corrected. A few centuries later, another Greek writer presented plague in *History of the Peloponnesian War*.[8] Thucydides chronicled the war between Athens and Sparta from 431 to 404 BCE while also serving as an Athenian general for a portion of the war. When he described the plague's arrival in the city of Athens, plague is clearly a disease and not just a "stroke or blow" as it was in *The Iliad*.

Thucydides reports that "the plague" appeared in Athens a few days after the Spartans (Peloponnesians) invaded that city. Although the plague affected other parts of the country, "there was no record of the disease being so virulent anywhere else or causing so many deaths as it did in Athens."[9] Plague is clearly a disease here in fifth-century Greece, but what disease was it exactly? From Thucydides' catalogue of symptoms, it resembles smallpox more than bubonic plague. Victims initially experienced some form of headache, inflamed eyes, and bleeding in the oral cavity. There were also upper respiratory symptoms, including sneezing, hoarseness, and coughing; these ailments were followed by gastrointestinal symptoms of nausea, vomiting, and abdominal pain. This symptomatology, however, could indicate any viral infection, including yellow fever, measles, typhoid, inhalational anthrax, and bubonic plague.[10]

But when Thucydides continues to chronicle the course of the illness over time, it strikingly resembles smallpox. Thucydides also comments on the survivors of the disease experiencing blindness. Michael Oldstone claims that smallpox caused blindness in some people who survived the disease in seventeenth- and eighteenth-century Europe.[11] Smallpox certainly was not alien to the ancient world. Oldstone considers, as other scientists have, that the Egyptian king Ramses V died from smallpox in 1157 BCE. This conclusion is based on the pustules found on the head and neck of his mummified body, which was discovered in the nineteenth century.[12]

Thucydides' detailed reporting of this disease that he calls "plague" in fifth-century Athens provides another definition for this word: an infectious disease causing great mortality; this definition of plague is also found in the *OED*. This disease in Thucydides' Greece certainly was infectious and accompanied by a high mortality rate. Many Athenian doctors contracted it, for example, due to their contact with the sick, and "many dead bodies [lay] about unburied."[13]

Thucydides, like Homer, offered sources for this plague as he chronicled the Athenians' views after the disease's outbreak. As these views are examined, we should keep in mind that Thucydides was an Athenian and he fought against the Spartans. Furthermore, there are no other records of a firsthand chronicle of the Peloponnesian War other than Thucydides' account. In other words, we do not have a Peloponnesian view of the war or the plague.

One view of the plague amongst Athenians was that it had a human source that was specifically Spartan:

> In the city of Athens it [the plague] appeared suddenly, and the first cases were among the population of Piraeus [a seaport town], where there were no wells at that time, so that it was supposed by them that the Peloponnesians had poisoned the reservoirs.[14]

The Athenian perception that the Spartans caused the plague in their town by poisoning the reservoirs hauntingly forecasts the fourteenth-century Europeans' perception that the Jews poisoned wells and therefore somehow caused bubonic plague. Here in Greece, the Athenians already were killing Spartans in their war and did not launch an unprovoked campaign of murder against their enemy as we will witness in fourteenth-century Europe. The enemy was the human source of plague in Thucydides' chronicle, but this enemy (the Spartans) could potentially contract the disease, whereas in Homer's poem Chryses and other Trojans were not in danger of suffering from Apollo's plague nor were they blamed for it.

In the above quoted passage, Thucydides offers a human source of plague that is really a matter of one social group (the Athenians) assigning blame for a disease to a different social group (the Spartans) who are their enemies at this time. In his introduction, Thucydides admits that it was the Athenian growth of power that provoked the Spartans into battle initially. The ancient Greeks did not know that smallpox was caused by a virus, nor could they prove that diseases are caused by a variety of microbes, including viruses, bacteria, parasites, and fungi. Perhaps it is not so odd that the dominant power under attack by a lesser power in Greece would attribute the microbial attack of plague to their enemy. Blaming the Spartans for plague may have served as the Athenian justification for continuing the war against them.

To Thucydides' credit, however, he did not endorse the Spartan enemy as the cause of plague, in spite of contracting the disease himself and recovering from it. After presenting the Athenian poisoning theory, Thucydides rationally explains that he cannot definitively determine the cause of plague, and he relieves himself of the responsibility of finding it by claiming that other writers may be able to discover it. Whether or not Thucydides' personal experience with the disease influenced his objectivity once he did recover, or he remained faithful to his earlier stated goal for this history to give a "factual reporting of the events of the war" and "not even to be guided by my own general impressions,"[15] he presents an Athenian view of disease but does not support that view. Thucydides' objectivity stands in contrast to several medieval chroniclers who not only endorse but also perpetuate Jewish sources of plague in the fourteenth century.

Homer's *The Iliad* and Thucydides' *History of the Peloponnesian War* represent early perceptions of plague in the Western culture. These perceptions are also found in the Old and New Testaments of the Bible, a book that has probably influenced future perceptions of plague more than any other written text due to its wide circulation and popularity among so many different religious groups. Representations of plague in the Old Testament, in particular, intersect with those in ancient Greece.

The Old and New Testaments of the Bible are viewed by many religious groups as sacred texts. They also can be treated, however, as historical documents and viewed through a secular lens with the purpose of exploring, as objectively as possible, two different religious groups' views of plague and the probable influence of these views on later Western cultures.

The Old Testament can be read as the earliest textual record of the Jewish people's perceptions of and relationship with a divine being. It also serves as the earliest record of this society's perceptions of plague. In the book of Genesis, the word *plague* is not specifically employed but it is implied when Pharaoh and the Egyptians are punished by God (the Jews' divine being) for Pharaoh's marriage to Abram's beautiful wife, Sara, upon their entrance into Egypt. This incident occurs in Genesis 12 when God initially asks this most reverent patriarch, Abram, to take his wife and his nephew, Lot, and travel into a land where God will make them "a great people."[16] God makes it clear to Abram that he will reward anyone who respects his family and punish anyone who does not exhibit this respect.

When Abram takes his family into Egypt because famine had enveloped the surrounding land they travel through, Abram's divine being punishes the Egyptians for exhibiting disrespect toward his family. Upon entering Egypt, Abram pretends to be Sara's sibling instead of her husband because he fears he will be killed for his beautiful wife. Even though the Egyptian Pharaoh does not know Sara is married when he marries her, "the Lord smote [him] and his court with great calamities, because of Abram's wife, Sarai."[17] These "great calamities" are not detailed in this passage but do not sound particularly beneficial for the Egyptians. The Lord's punishment ("smote") of a group that violated a devout follower's marital relationship resembles the "stroke or blow" of burning arrows that Apollo wielded against the Greek army in *The Iliad* for its violation of the daughter of his devotee. The calamities cease for the Egyptians, as they did for the Greeks in Homer's poem, when they correct their behavior and safely return Sara to Abram.

Plague as a form of divine punishment for another social group's violation of a Jewish religious value is more pronounced in 1 Kings. This disease certainly resembles *Yersinia pestis* and it is wielded by the Jewish divine being against the Philistines because of their disrespect and disregard for the symbol of the covenant made between God and the Jews. In 1 Kings 4–5, the Israelites are engaged in a losing battle with the Philistines who subsequently steal the ark of God, or the Ark of the Covenant. This ark is the tabernacle built by Jews upon Moses' return from receiving the Ten Commandments from God on Mount Sinai. This tabernacle serves as the symbol of God's covenant with Moses and the Jewish community; if they follow these commandments, their divine being will protect them.

The book of 1 Kings is told from a Jewish perspective because the symbol of the Jewish community's relationship with its divine being is valued above the Philistine's relationship with their own god. When the Philistines pilfer the Ark of the Covenant and place it before Dagon, a statue of their divine being, it falls. More significantly, the Philistines are punished with plague by the Jewish divine being for their violation:

> And now the Lord sent a heavy plague on the men of Azotus [the Philistines] and its neighbourhood, to their undoing, a plague of swellings in the groin. All through their townships, all over the country-side, the infection spread; the mice, too, swarmed every-where; in the city, the dead lay piled in heaps.[18]

This description of plague captures its different meanings: Plague is a "stroke or blow" as it is wielded by the Lord; it is an infectious disease with a high mortality rate as it "spread" and "swarmed everywhere," producing "heaps" of dead bodies; and it is a divine punishment for a social group (the Philistines) that did not respect the religious values of the favored society in this story. This plague ends when the Philistines eventually correct their behavior by returning the Ark of the Covenant to the Israelites.

The actual disease described in this passage is worth looking at more closely because it provides some insight into the possible age of the *Yersinia* bacterium and its *plague* label. The "swellings in the groin" experienced by the Philistines suggest the buboes, or swollen lymph glands of *Yersinia* infection. The rapidity of transmission ("all through their townships, all over the country-side") suggests this infection, as does the vector of transmission: "the mice, too, swarmed everywhere." Although the rat flea, *Xenopsylla cheopis*, is the most common carrier of the bacterium to humans, this flea also can live in other rodent populations, including mice, as we still experience today in the southwestern region of the United States.[19] This biblical passage suggests that *Yersinia* infection perhaps was extant before the Common Era.

Plague also appears in the New Testament of the Bible, which includes the Gospels of Matthew, Mark, Luke, and John, as well as epistles from Jesus' other followers, and concludes with the book of the Apocalypse or Revelations, as it is commonly referred to today. The Apocalypse is the apostle John's vision of the end of the world that he claims to have received from Jesus in a trance-like state. This text is notable for its detailed descriptions of the Christian schema of the slow destruction of life on earth and the eventual divine creation of the eternal city, the New Jerusalem, where Jesus' followers will peacefully live forever with their divine being. John's destructive vision in this text may have been influenced by the Roman persecution of the Christian community as he wrote it. But this New Testament book has been greatly revered by many Christian sects over time, including our own, as an actual forecast of events that will usher in eternity.

According to John's vision, humans on earth, Christians and non-Christians alike, will be "test[ed]"[20] in this move toward the end of the world. John does not detail the exact deeds one will need to perform in order to pass this "test" to gain a place in what he terms "the Lamb's book of life,"[21] or the guaranteed portal of entry into the eternal city of the New Jerusalem. It is assumed, however, throughout the book of the Apocalypse that followers of Jesus need to remain steadfast in their devotion, in spite of the enormous ecological catastrophes they will endure during the long destruction of the earth. This message is indicated by a flying angel who bellows to humans who already have experienced famine and fire: "Fear the Lord, he cried aloud, and give him the praise; the hour of his judgment has come."[22] The reminder to remain steadfast in praising ("fearing") this divine being is not restricted to Christians; the angel delivers this message "to every race and tribe and language and people."[23] The angel seems to be inciting other religious groups to convert to Christianity in order to be saved ultimately by this divine being: people should continue to praise God, who is primarily manifested as Jesus throughout this book, even while they are enduring this suffering.

Plague is responsible for a significant amount of the suffering and destruction that humans are supposed to endure in John's vision. In other words, plague is part of the "test" for salvation. The source of plague in this New Testament book is definitively divine as it is in the Old Testament passages we examined. While in the Old Testament plague is sent by a divine being to punish the behavior of a social group that already violated the relationship between the Jewish community and its divine being, here plague is a type of preemptive corrective for those people who will not worship this Christian divine being in the future. John's book is a vision of what is supposed to happen, not a record of what has happened or is happening. For example, when Jesus will hold a scroll with seven seals in heaven and the seventh seal is to be broken by him, countless numbers of horses and riders will be unleashed to follow the four angels who have been awaiting the time to destroy a portion of humankind. These horses in their purposeful trot emit destruction from their mouths that "were three plagues, from which a third part of mankind perished."[24] John continues to reveal that the surviving remainder of humankind "still worshipped evil spirits, false gods of gold and silver."[25] Plague will destroy anyone who worships divine beings other than the Christian one with the implication that if one foregoes this type of "false" worship, he or she may be saved from such a plague in the future.

The threat of plague is further extended to those people who actually worship Satan, or as John calls them "the men who bore the beast's mark, and worshipped his image."[26] Seven angels, to be exact, will carry plagues in cups which are "those last plagues by which the vengeance of God is finally achieved."[27] Plague is the vessel of divine punishment. These seven plagues in Apocalypse 16 primarily are not diseases, but calamities intended to harm disbelievers, especially Satan worshippers. The first plague poured out of the cup by one of the seven angels onto the earth causes a malignant ulcer upon those who carry this supposed mark of the beast. This ulcer seems designed to cause pain as opposed to just illness. The third plague is not a disease either, as it turns the rivers into blood, but this blood is a boon for devout worshippers of the Christian divine being.[28] Some of the remaining seven plagues include intensifying the heat of the sun, turning Satan's kingdom to darkness, and obliterating the Euphrates River. The final plague disrupts the earth's foundation with "a violent earthquake" and paves the way for the construction of the eternal city.[29]

Earlier in John's text, he intimates that plague is a disease when the fourth seal of the scroll is broken by Jesus and the figure of Death rides a horse killing humans "by the sword, by famine, by plague."[30] Since plague is distinct here from violence and famine it could mean a disease; however, this disease is not specifically characterized and is never mentioned again in this book. The Christian perspective presented in this New Testament book portrays plague instead as a long series of ecological calamities that are imposed upon humankind by a divine being in order to correct and prevent future violations of the Christian belief system, in particular the persistent worship of what Christians view as false gods. Plague is a divine corrective for behavior that violates, or more accurately *will* violate, this particular religious group's belief system.

This review of early written Western thoughts about *plague*, with consideration of the *OED*, produces a definition for this word that will navigate us through different centuries. Plague is an affliction usually bestowed by a particular social or religious group's notion of a divine being that causes pain, prolonged suffering, and even death. Plague often serves as a corrective for certain behaviors that violate some aspect of a particular belief system. When a disease is called a plague, it is usually highly infectious and accompanied by a high mortality rate as seen with smallpox and *Yersinia* infection. As a disease, plague is often assigned a divine cause by a particular group of people; when a specific human cause is assigned, the process of scapegoating is underway as seen most notably with fourteenth-century bubonic plague and later in the twentieth century with AIDS.

PART II

Bubonic Plague

CHAPTER 3

Fourteenth-Century Europe

Stephen lay in his Room 304 bed around 3 P.M. on a serene spring day in 1989. The year 1989 would close with 23,500 AIDS-related deaths.[1] It seemed like we wrapped a dead body every night. I guess we did. Stephen's dark and groomed wavy hair was a sign of his fastidiousness in caring for his 30-something appearance. It was only a sign at this point because there was not one inch of his skin left unmarred by the purplish lesions; his face was particularly marked and swollen. Stephen was not a model but the photographs surrounding him of happier days before his illness belied this fact.

I was not surprised by Stephen's reaction to his Kaposi's sarcoma (KS)—an AIDS-related cancer and opportunistic infection now known to be caused by the human herpes simplex 8 virus. He had withdrawn from the world. The pervasive admiration for his physical beauty that he was accustomed to receiving from people he met in clubs, at parties, and as he walked up Madison Avenue to work had silently faded.

Stephen's infectious disease doctor, Dr. G, arrived on the unit to discuss possible treatment options for his aggressive KS. Some of the lesions that smothered the surface area of his skin were large enough, especially around his groin, to conjure up images of buboes, even though none of us, including his doctor, had actually cared for a patient with bubonic plague. These lesions were the visible stigmata of his deadly cancer that now infiltrated his lungs. His worsening cough produced frothy, bloody sputum.

When Dr. G left his room, I asked him how Stephen responded to his treatment options. He could receive some fairly toxic chemotherapy and maybe some radiation, but nothing would stop the HIV from invading his T helper cells, the ultimate reason for his slow and gruesome death from this cancer. It was obvious that the doctor was pained by Stephen's disfigured appearance and imminent death. "He looks like he has bubonic plague. It's as if each lesion represents every sexual partner he ever had." I said, "Well, he must have had a hell of a lot of them." I was fairly positive that Dr. G was not casting judgment on Stephen's behavior as our conversation continued, nor was I; rather, he was attempting to understand what prompted this unusually handsome man to engage in sexual intercourse, as Stephen admitted, sometimes up to four times a day. "A healthy libido," was my somewhat sarcastic response to his query.

Images of bubonic plague flourished in our minds during this time period, especially when caring for patients with such pronounced KS lesions like Stephen had. The connection that Dr. G drew between Stephen's multiple lesions and his sexual partners in the context of plague illustrates that even the most devoted and compassionate health-care workers were influenced by the plague mentality that enveloped AIDS. More specific origins of this mentality can be found in the dusty accounts of bubonic plague's most dire debut in fourteenth-century Europe.

The first pandemic of plague extended out of Egypt and into Europe and Asia Minor in 541 CE with recurrences over the next 200 years. The second pandemic began in 1346 and recurred until the early 1700s. This pandemic has been referred to by historians and medical scientists as "the greatest biomedical disaster" and "public health disaster" in history.[2] The 1346 plague was indeed a disaster with huge population losses, especially throughout Europe. We are fortunate to have so much written material that records the disastrous effects of the disease.

Historical certainty regarding the actual number of deaths from the disease during the 1346 outbreak probably will never be attained. It was difficult in the fourteenth century to collect and record taxes from remote families and villages, which had been a means for tracking the census. Furthermore, the swiftness and large number of deaths from the illness made it difficult for officials to record every dead body. A recent historian analyzed tax- and rent-paying households throughout Europe before and after the 1346 plague and estimated that prior to the disease eighty million people comprised the European population and in its aftermath a few years later only thirty million people remained.[3]

The Crimean seaport Kaffa has been targeted by historians as the epicenter of the 1346 plague. Italian merchants conducting business there contracted the disease and carried it with them back to Italy while infecting other seaport towns like Alexandria along the way. In the autumn of 1347, Alexandria experienced 100–200 deaths daily and by the following spring that number increased to 1,000 per day.[4] When the disease-carrying vessels arrived back home in Messina, Sicily, in July 1347, it was not long before the plague enveloped the country. Boccaccio—the Italian author most famous for *The*

Decameron, a collection of 100 tales told by fictional female and male nobles as they journey to the countryside to escape plague—discussed the devastating reality of the disease and proposed that more than 100,000 people perished in Florence alone.[5] He lamented how "great a number of splendid palaces, fine houses, and noble dwellings . . . were bereft of all who had lived there, down to the tiniest child!"[6] The author might have exaggerated in his proposal of the number of the dead, although historians estimate a population loss of 55–65 percent in Florence, but he certainly witnessed death on an unimaginable scale.[7] Most of the writers who lived through this pandemic were prone to hyperbolic descriptions of events but this is better than no account at all. This was the first pandemic of plague that produced a "continuous succession of literary and historical records,"[8] especially in Italy and England, and these records are invaluable as a window to a world struggling to cope with and understand an infectious disease with a high mortality rate.

From Italy, the plague spread to Africa and the Iberian Peninsula, where 65 percent of the Spanish population perished.[9] By the summer of 1348, the plague raged in Paris and 500 people died every day, according to one medieval chronicler.[10] As it spread throughout the country, even the English king's daughter, Princess Joan, fatally encountered it in Bordeaux on her way to marry the prince of Castille. By the end of that summer, the plague traveled to England with merchant sailors who docked in Bristol. The fourteenth-century chronicler, Henry Knighton, claimed that almost everyone died in that town.[11] Some modern historians place the death toll for England at half of the population within two years after the disease's arrival.[12]

The clinical course of the fourteenth-century disease correlated with that of *Yersinia pestis* infection, even today. One of the first chroniclers of 1346 plague, the Italian Gabriele de' Mussis, reported that at first a "chilly stiffness" seizes the body and then a "hard, solid boil" erupts in the armpit or groin region. The next stage involves fever and headaches. Some people vomit blood and become prostrate. Death can occur the day symptoms arise but usually it is delayed for three to five days. The chance of recovery is slim if vomiting of blood occurs but possible if only the boil and fever are present.[13] The English chronicler John of Reading briefly described the "ulcers" that occurred in the armpits or groin with death following three days later.[14]

There are three types of *Yersinia* infection still referred to as plague by the medical community today. Bubonic plague infects the lymph nodes; septicemic plague infects the blood; and pneumonic plague infects the lungs. The incubation period for all types of plague is two to eight days (this is the time from exposure to the bacterium until the onset of symptoms). The presentation of symptoms today is similar to Mussis' description in 1346: fever and chills. The temperature can go as high as 104 degrees Fahrenheit as was witnessed in a New Mexico man who traveled to New York City in 2002 and was diagnosed with the plague.[15] Headache, prostration—even delirium—and the classic bubo (a swollen, tender lymph node in the armpit or groin that appears blackish) follow the high fevers. If the infection enters the bloodstream, it becomes septicemic, and if it enters the lungs it becomes pneumonic. Pneumonic plague is the only form that can be directly transmitted between humans when infected droplets carry the bacterium through coughing. Mussis' description of the vomiting of blood could be the expectoration of bloody sputum seen in the pneumonic form of the disease. If left untreated, plague today has a fourteenth-century-like mortality rate of 50–60 percent, especially the septicemic and pneumonic forms.[16] But thanks to the discovery of antibiotics in the twentieth century, streptomycin and tetracycline readily treat and cure this bacterial infection.

The fourteenth-century world did not know that plague is transmitted by fleas—primarily *Xenopsylla cheopis* and *Pulex irritans*—that feed on rats.[17] These infected fleas can survive up to 80 days without their rat host before they bite humans and transmit the *Yersinia pestis* bacterium that causes the disease.[18] Fleas, not humans, are the primary vector of transmission. But in the fourteenth century, the human senses were offered as a vector of transmission. John Clynn, an Irish chronicler, reported that 14,000 people died in Dublin during the pandemic and he claimed that "touching" the dead or the sick transmitted the disease.[19] Clynn might not have been that far off the mark with his supposition, considering that the living caring for the dead and the sick could have been bitten by nearby infected fleas, or contact with infected bodily fluids in the sick or dead was the source of transmission. One microbiologist thinks that Christians who cleared the dead bodies catapulted by Tartars into the city walls of Kaffa during the 1346 outbreak there contracted the disease after touching them.[20]

Other writers attributed the transmission of plague primarily to sight. The Italian chronicler Mussis thought that one person could "infect people and places with this disease by look alone," a supposition that certainly characterizes the extreme contagiousness of plague.[21] When the plague reached Siena, Italy, Agnola di Tura's poignant description of the panic surrounding its arrival also contained a theory of sensory transmission: "Father abandoned child, wife husband, one brother another; for this illness seemed to strike through the breath and sight."[22] Even medieval physicians attributed the disease's deadly spread to sight. A Montpellier physician who wrote a treatise on plague in 1349 described it as a "visible vapour" contracted through sight.[23] Pope Clement VI's personal physician, the surgeon Gui de Chauliac, commented on what appears to be the pneumonic form of plague and theorized that living together in close quarters with the sick as well as "merely through looking, one person caught it from the other."[24]

Modern medical science proves that so-called plague and other infectious diseases are not and have not been transmitted through sight. But there has been doubt in scientific circles over the past few decades regarding the etiology of the disease referred to as plague in fourteenth-century Europe. In 1985, zoologist Graham Twigg questioned that the fourteenth-century pandemic was bubonic plague (*Yersinia pestis* infection) based on the lack of evidence for a substantial population of dead rats. According to Twigg, huge rat mortalities would have been necessary in the Middle Ages as the precipitating event for a plague outbreak in humans. Fleas carry the *Yersinia* bacterium and infect rats, especially the black rat *(Rattus rattus)*, which then die; subsequently, the fleas search for new hosts (humans) only after their primary hosts (rats) are unavailable. Twigg finds it curious that medieval writers did not mention a large number of rat corpses before and during the 1346 pandemic, but he admits that "rats were so much a part of everyday life as to be taken for granted."[25] Perhaps medieval writers saw no reason to mention their quite familiar long-tailed companions. This lacuna in the writings, however, opens the door for Twigg to search for another disease as the culprit: anthrax, in particular pulmonary anthrax. The anthrax bacillus is "much hardier and more versatile than *Yersinia pestis*."[26] This organism could have survived the climatic changes in the fourteenth century, classified by some scientists as the "Little Ice Age."[27] Anthrax does not rely on fleas or rats for its own survival, rather it lives in the soil where livestock, such as sheep and cattle, contract it; subsequent transmission occurs through touching or eating the infected animals or inhaling the bacillus from close contact with the soil.

Murrain (anthrax in animals) has been documented in the fourteenth century, and Norman Cantor mentions that excavations carried out in 1989 near Edinburgh, Scotland, revealed anthrax spores.[28] The symptoms of pulmonary anthrax—bloody sputum, difficulty in breathing, high temperature, and even blue skin—as well as the death that occurs within two to three days from the onset of symptoms are similar to pneumonic plague symptoms. Twigg argues throughout his study that the swift rate of transmission of the disease in the fourteenth century is more characteristic of pulmonary anthrax than any type of plague.

Other historians uphold the accepted view that bubonic plague was the disease that swept Europe in the mid-fourteenth century. Benedictow, for example, presents scientific evidence for the skeletal remains of the black rat throughout Europe dating back to the Roman occupation and extending through the medieval period.[29] If the black rat was there, bubonic plague was not far behind. In addition, John Kelly presents DNA evidence of the presence of *Yersinia pestis* at medieval plague burial sites, including that found by French paleomicrobiologists in the dental pulp of corpses in fourteenth-century southern France.[30]

Perhaps one solution for the debate over the disease culprit is Norman Cantor's proposal that *both* bubonic plague and anthrax coexisted during the fourteenth century pandemic.[31] The evidence still seems to lean more toward bubonic plague; but whether or not the *Yersinia* or the anthrax bacillus was responsible for the massive mortality rates in fourteenth-century Europe, this world viewed the disease as *plague*. Both illnesses do fulfill one of the definitions I have offered for plague: a highly infectious disease that causes a great mortality.

Lacking the benefits of later medical knowledge, especially nineteenth-century germ theory—in particular Koch's postulates designed to prove that a particular organism causes a particular disease—fourteenth-century writers described the disease that killed their family, friends, and neighbors primarily as *pestilence,* one of plague's synonyms. In England, Middle English—a blend of Germanic English and French—was spoken in this century. *Pláge* was the Middle English word for *plague* derived from the Old French language,[32] but its usage was not popular in the fourteenth century except in Scandinavian countries.[33] This Nordic usage entered England sometime in the fifteenth century.

Instead, *pestilence* was used frequently by English writers to describe the 1348 pandemic. One chronicler described the introduction of the disease into England as "the seeds of the terrible pestilence" carried by a sailor from Gascony.[34] These chroniclers wrote in Latin and we are served by a modern English translation here, but authors writing about plague in their vernacular language later in this century still referred to it as *pestilence.* For instance, William Langland's book-length poem *Piers the Plowman* contains these references to the disease.[35] This poem was written around 1377 in alliterative Middle English, a dialect spoken in the northwest region, and it is a dream vision. The poet repeatedly falls asleep and dreams. In these dreams, Will meets personified characters such as the Seven Deadly Sins who are responsible for the populace's pervasive turn away from the Catholic Church and ultimately from salvation. Other characters such as Reason and Wit try to lead these supposedly fallen people toward the plowman, Piers, who alone knows the way to salvation. I admit that even the most dedicated English literature majors remain daunted by the subject matter and length of this poem, but it serves as a social commentary on religious and class relations, their attendant values, and the consequences of violating these values. For example, early in the poem Reason preaches to the people, including the king, that plague is a consequence of sin: "He preached that these pestilences [were] for pure sin."[36]

Langland may have had the great pestilence of 1348 in mind here or the second wave of the epidemic in 1361 that resulted in a 20 percent mortality for the country.

Geoffrey Chaucer, the most popular medieval English writer, referred to the fourteenth-century disease as *pestilence* at moments in *The Canterbury Tales*, which he did not begin to write until the late 1380s, well after the most severe plague outbreaks.[37] This ambitious work remains incomplete due to the author's death in 1400, but the 24 fictional tales we do have are told by a socially diverse cast of characters who range from the aristocratic knight and monk to the middle-class merchant and cloth maker, the Wife of Bath, and to a humble preacher, the Parson. Like Boccaccio's *The Decameron*, Chaucer's tales are a fictional journey; however, his 29 pilgrims are traveling from London to Canterbury in order to pay homage to the martyred Saint Thomas á Becket, the archbishop of the late twelfth century who was killed in his own church by King Henry II's noble followers.

Chaucer did not devote time to describe the plague like Boccaccio, but the few references to it illustrate the disease's continual impact on the popular imagination as this century progressed. The Wife of Bath concludes her tale, an Arthurian romance that serves her untimely feminist vision that wives should have the ultimate power in their marriages, with a prayer to Jesus to wield plague as a punishment. She asks him to send a "true pestilence"[38] to misery old men like her previous husband who would not give her control of the household finances. This radical character subverts her society's prevalent view that plague is a divine punishment for unorthodox behavior by praying for the disease to correct this quite accepted behavior of husbands.

In "The Pardoner's Tale," Chaucer has his Pardoner ironically narrate a story about the consequences of following greed. Pardoners sold saints' relics and other religious talismans in exchange for pardoning people's sins. Pardoners could make quite a profit in this ostensibly altruistic line of work, and Chaucer's pilgrim has no problem working the crowd during the pilgrimage. The tale is set in Flanders during an active plague outbreak and we meet three friends drinking and conversing in a tavern. Outside a bell rings indicating the journey of yet another corpse to the grave. A young boy who is present explains that the dead man was their friend and he is merely one among "a thousand [who have been] slain [by] this pestilence," which has especially decimated the village a mile away.[39] Although this tale is set in continental Flanders, Chaucer employs the popular English reference to plague as *pestilence*.

Continental medieval writers expressed their society's perception of the disease as both *plague* and *pestilence*. An Austrian chronicler in 1348 described the fire that fell from the sky producing smoke that contained the "pestilence," and "the deadly plague" was so pervasive that many cities locked their gates to prevent the looting of the dead's property.[40] The monks who wrote the *Great Chronicle of France* recorded the disease's arrival there as "the plague," which they claimed killed 800 people a day in Paris. These monks also described the disease as "pestilence" when they observed people dancing in a town in an effort to ward it off.[41]

Boccaccio alternated between calling the disease "the recent plague" and "this pestilence." At one point he even labeled the disease a "scourge" when he described uninfected people's abandonment of sick family members, even children, as a result of their extreme fear of contagion.[42] *Scourge* was an extant term in the Middle Ages that meant a whip or slash used for punishment.[43] Boccaccio's use of this synonym for plague indicates that this world certainly viewed the highly infectious disease as a punishment. The usage of this word also has persisted in twenty-first-century references to AIDS. During a presidential debate in the summer of 2007 between Democratic presidential nominee candidates, a panelist prefaced one of her questions with a report that 69 percent of HIV positive people in America are African Americans. She then asked the candidates what they will do to fight this "scourge."[44] Without yet examining the genesis of AIDS' construction as a plague, we can perhaps appreciate the detrimental connotation of employing this plague synonym.

Astrological and divine explanations for plague were the primary ones offered by fourteenth-century Europeans in an effort to understand and control its devastation. In October 1348, the Paris Medical Faculty issued a monograph on the causes of and treatments for plague. They proposed that on March 20, 1345, "the conjunction of three planets in Aquarius" produced the polluted air that carried the disease. In particular, the faculty used Aristotle's theory about Saturn and Jupiter conjoining and producing diseases on earth. As the Faculty examined more immediate causes, they reiterated that "corrupted air" gave rise to the plague.[45] A southern Austrian chronicler similarly proposed that a fire that fell from heaven in the Far East produced a smoke that carried the pestilence.[46]

In England, Chaucer wrote about the astrological influence on plague in "The Knight's Tale." This romantic tale, set in ancient Athens, focuses on two knights vying for the love of the same woman. They encounter obstacles over many years that prevent each of them from being near her, and when they finally are they have to joust in order to win her heart. Before the battle, one of the knights visits the temple of Venus to pray for success and the other knight prays to Mars. As Venus and Mars quarrel over the mortal winner, Saturn, Venus' father, interjects by detailing his own history of power in mortal affairs. One of his credentials is "the father of pestilence."[47] Although

Saturn is an anthropomorphized ancient Greek god here, Chaucer expressed the fourteenth-century view that this planet was associated with plague. Medieval thoughts about the influence of planets and the Earth's atmosphere on the emergence of diseases move toward a scientific, or at least a pseudoscientific, theory of disease etiology. But this type of theory was not the predominant one in the fourteenth century. Boccaccio, who clearly accepted the planetary causality of plague, also presented a divine one: "it was punishment signifying God's righteous anger at our iniquitous way of life."[48] The Italian historian Gabriele de' Mussis presented a strong case for a divine cause of plague in his chronicle. There he creates a conversation between God and the earth that focuses on humans' sins offending God. He has God announce the solution for this offence: "I bring retribution giving each individual his due."[49] This retribution is primarily plague. The reported conversation between God and humans does not contain the caveat that it is a fictional dialogue employed by the historian to explain plague's arrival. Mussis attempted to make a divine cause of plague factual.

What exactly were the iniquities or sins that could have provoked such an extreme punishment by God in the medieval mind? In general, medieval European society was gripped by a Christian belief system, mainly Catholicism, which was hard to escape, considering the Catholic Church also held an amazing amount of political power. In England, for example, higher levels of the clergy held political office and a good amount of land as feudal lords, which gave them votes in parliament. Governmental decisions and laws were influenced by Catholicism. Christian ideology certainly circulated outside of the walls of the Church. The populace accepted the idea that God inflicted plague as a punishment for anyone who violated Christian values, namely anyone who committed one of the seven deadly sins or any minor vice that flows from them. An anonymous fourteenth-century English poem, "On the Pestilence," begins by asking why the plague has killed so many people. The answer offered by the poet is: "Because vices rule unchallenged here."[50] Specific sins are listed throughout the poem such as the sloth of shepherds in tending their flocks, the rich exploiting the poor, and women overstepping their assigned gender roles.

Similarly, an English treatise on pestilence written in the 1360s explained why so many children perished during the 1361 epidemic: "and it may be that it is in vengeance of this sin of dishonouring and despising fathers and mothers that God is slaying children by pestilence."[51] Plague was viewed also as a corrective for unfavorable behavior. Thomas Brinton preached during the 1360s in England that children's death from plague was "designed by God to jolt their families and friends into good behavior."[52] Imagine the poor children who practiced these admonitions and contracted the illness anyway, and those surviving families who were influenced to view their offspring's death as a reminder of their own supposed "bad" behavior.

By the summer of 1349 in Tournai, France, the Town Council was so desperate to halt the 5–15 daily deaths from plague that they surmised this divine vengeance could be thwarted by raising the morality of the town's inhabitants. One of the town's orders advised unmarried, cohabitating men and women to marry immediately in an effort to avert more plague deaths.[53] Back in England, the chronicler John of Reading recorded extramarital sexual intercourse as one cause of the pestilence in 1365.[54]

Medieval European society in general was socially arranged in a strict hierarchy with nobles and wealthy churchmen at the top; a growing class of merchants, small business owners, and independent landholders in the middle; and the peasantry and paid laborers at the bottom. People believed this social structure was divinely ordained because the Church said it was: One's social class was given by God like one's hair color. Any sign of social activity not befitting one's social ranking was viewed as a sin, and during plague outbreaks these social transgressions were offered as a cause of divine punishment.

In England, peasants under the servitude of a feudal lord were not paid for their work in cash. Some of them took the opportunity to engage in labor they were paid for elsewhere. With the massive loss in population during the 1348 epidemic, surviving workers were able to command even higher wages for their labor since there were fewer workers to go around. King Edward III and parliament did not take this elevation in income lightly, and in 1349 they issued labor laws that would return the wages of these lower-class workers to preplague rates. These workers, however, did not comply with the new laws; they did not have to, after all, since their labor services were in high demand. The king issued a letter to the bishops urging them to correct the workers' "sinfulness and pride . . . so that merciful God might repel the plague and illness."[55] Low-born workers who performed an activity (wage labor) that potentially could raise them to a higher social ranking were deemed sinful and therefore as contributors to God's punishment of the country with plague.

In *Piers the Plowman*, Langland referred to another social behavior that was deemed sinful: the growing materialism consuming all ranks of English society. The higher wages steadily earned by the lower classes enabled them to buy more goods, such as meat and finer clothing, while wealthier people continued to indulge in the goods of their choice. Langland expresses the popular view that fixating on goods constituted the sin of pride. Furthermore, this materialistic focus has diverted attention away from serious religious devotion with plague as the consequence: "so has pride grown/ . . . /that prayers have no power to stop the pestilence."[56]

Indulgence in certain types of fashion was also viewed as a sin that indirectly provoked this divine punishment on English society. John of Reading commented on the new style of clothing adopted in the 1360s. Apparently these garments were more revealing than they hitherto had been as they "failed to conceal their arses or their private parts."[57] Ultimately, this provocative clothing prevented people from kneeling in church to praise God and the saints, as Reading reports, and this lack of reverence was thought to cause the plague.

This highly religious European society, however, was not above assigning blame to its own church for the plague. Mussis in Italy attributed priests' neglect in their congregational duties as one incitement for plague.[58] He explained in his feigned conversation between God and humans that when priests do not educate their followers and encourage them to repent, sin ensues and God's punishment with plague follows. This diverted attention of priests from their congregations was in part due to their own interest in the wealth they acquired through land and salaries. Chaucer's description of his monk in *The Canterbury Tales* highlights the worldly indulgences of the clergy that kept them from devoting more time to their congregations.[59] This monk hunts—a popular noble past time in the Middle Ages—the sleeves of his habit are lined with fur, a gold pin fastens his hood, and he loves to dine on voluptuous swans. John of Reading, the English historian, attributed this kind of "superfluous finery" worn by monks like Chaucer's who had taken vows of poverty as another provocation for divine punishment in the form of plague.[60]

European society in the fourteenth century viewed disobedience, sexual indiscretions, social advancement, and secular and ecclesiastical materialism as sins that ultimately caused the plague. This society had little doubt about their Christian divine being's role in this disease. After all, Dr. Alexandre Yersin's discovery of the bacterium that causes so-called plague was still 500 years away.

But there were other medieval Europeans who did not turn to the heavens searching for causes of plague but instead fabricated a human cause: the Jews. The devastating mortality rates and suffering from this disease in the fourteenth century produced a variety of powerful reactions in the survivors. Some of these reactions coupled with a fairly pervasive anti-Semitism resulted in certain segments of the ruling Christian society blaming the Jews for the disease.

Despair is an expected reaction to watching a disease carry away so many family members, loved ones, and friends. As the Italian chronicler Agnolo di Tura objectively reports that he buried his own five children, he cannot help indulging in the universal despair of the survivors: "there was no one who wept for any death, for all awaited death."[61] The Italian poet Francesco Petrarch expressed his deflated sense of any connection with the world in the first poem that he wrote after his beloved Laura's death from plague in April 1348. The poem's title, "The Triumph of Death," indicates Petrarch's defeat by plague. It is a fine example of the lyrical dirges for which Petrarch was so famous, and this line captures his despair: "Virtue is dead; and dead is beauty too."[62]

The Canzoniere is Petrarch's lifetime collection of poems, including his sonnets. His love for Laura and his abject sorrow after her death from the plague are the main subjects of this collection. Petrarch might have had a particularly despairing reaction to Laura's death because he never really felt her love reciprocated, as far as we know. When Petrarch first met Laura in Avignon in April 1327, she was married to Hugues de Sade, an ancestor of the eighteenth-century Marquis de Sade. Her marriage, however, certainly did not impede Petrarch's intense feelings of love and loss when she perished during the 1348 epidemic. In Sonnet 310, for example, the description of a serene spring day with the natural elements themselves on the verge of falling in love quickly turns to bleakness as her death is recalled.[63]

Laura was not the only loved one Petrarch lost to the plague. During the 1361 outbreak in Milan, he lost his friends and his own son. In a letter written to his fellow poet and friend, Boccaccio, in 1363 his utter despondency from plague deaths was apparent as he wrote, "Of all my friends, only you remain."[64]

Italian reactions of despair to the plague were not unique. In the British Isles in the spring of 1349, Ieuan Gethin, a Welsh poet, described the disease as a ubiquitous and nebulous entity that was impossible to escape. "Death" enters his community "like [a] black smoke." It is "a plague" and "a rootless phantom" showing "no mercy."[65] Gethin's despair was particularly attributable to the fact that this description of plague was written after the herald of his own inevitable death appeared: the bubo under his arm.

A few decades after Gethin's reaction of despair to the plague, Chaucer wrote a poem, "The Book of the Duchess," to commemorate the death of the Duchess of Lancaster, Blanche, who died from plague in the late 1360s. Although plague is never specifically mentioned in this dream vision poem, sadness and extreme despair permeate the insomniac narrator's worldview. For instance, he has "feeling in nothing" as the poem begins.[66] The dark-cladded knight whom the narrator meets in his dream shares the narrator's weltanschauung when he explains: "This is my pain without remedy,/Always dying and I am not dead."[67] Eventually, in the conversation with the narrator during the dream the knight reveals that the cause of his extreme pain and despair is his wife's death. We cannot help but think that plague was the culprit of her death, and the knight's and even the narrator's despair.

Another reaction to plague in the fourteenth century was hedonism, the opposite of despair. Indulging excessively in one's desires was not necessarily gratuitous but was practiced by several Europeans as a method for preventing plague's arrival at their own doorstep. Boccaccio described that some people wanted to "ward off this appalling evil" through excessive drinking, singing, and a general disregard for the serious nature of the disease.[68] Similarly, two monks found people singing and dancing upon their entrance into the town of Saint-Denis, France, during the outbreak that was recorded in the *Great Chronicle of France*. The townspeople there explained: "we hope that our merrymaking will keep it away, and this is why we are dancing."[69] On the other hand, there were Europeans, like those described by an Austrian chronicler in 1348, who did not practice hedonism as a prophylactic but simply drank a lot of wine and committed random, violent beatings as a way of forgetting the tragic effects of the disease.[70]

Although despair and hedonism occupy the opposite ends of an emotional reaction plane—despair looks like sadness and hedonism looks like glee—both involve a certain degree of self-absorption. Despair is an excessive indulgence in pain and loss, and hedonism is an excessive indulgence in expressing and fulfilling pleasurable desires. The individualistic focus of these reactions does not readily lead to searching for a human cause of the disease, but fear of the disease and death could lead to scapegoating.

Fear is certainly an expected reaction to a highly infectious disease that killed more than half of the medieval European population. A Russian chronicler in 1352 recorded "severe epidemics" in several towns that produced "great fear and trepidation in all human beings. In Glukhov, at that time not a single human being was left, all were dead."[71] It is unlikely that everyone died in this town, but this type of dramatic statement was made frequently by medieval historians and illustrates the personal devastation of the authors as well as the fourteenth-century movement toward what Cantor calls a "death culture."[72] People became more focused on death, even becoming obsessed at times. Death became a popular subject in art and literature, as medieval poetry attests, because of plague.

In addition, death was viewed more as "a thing of horror" than as a peaceful passing as the century progressed,[73] and this view surfaces in cultural depictions of death. For example, the dance macabre (dance of death) occupied space in many paintings. This dance captures the fear of death and the mortal inability to control it as skeletons were commonly depicted dancing around humans in a mocking manner. One was found on the walls in the churchyard of the Innocents at Paris dated 1434.[74]

Not surprisingly, a fear of contagion was a part of this death culture. Boccaccio actually passed some judgment on this reaction in healthy survivors to the diseased victims: "they took a single and very inhuman precaution, namely to avoid or run away from the sick and their belongings, by which means they all thought that their own health would be preserved."[75] A bit of self-protection runs through the desire to flee here. Too much time with the victim indeed could result in transmission of the disease and one's own death, but total abandonment of the patient, impelled by fear, turns the plague victim all too easily into an object of disdain. Even physicians could not overcome this fear of contagion. Gui de Chauliac, the pope's doctor, felt "shameful for the physicians, who could give no help at all, especially as, out of fear of infection, they hesitated to visit the sick."[76]

Boccaccio actually thought that some of the neglected plague victims could have survived with care from doctors and family members.[77] Unfortunately, there was no effective medical treatment or cure for the plague in the fourteenth century. The treatises that were written offered prophylactic advice such as avoiding odoriferous smells by burning certain woods. Some people held handkerchiefs filled with strong herbs to their noses. In later centuries, plague doctors, hired by local towns and boards of health to treat victims of the disease throughout Europe, wore long-beaked masks filled with herbal sacks as they made their rounds of the sick. Unbeknownst to the people who wore respiratory barriers of any kind, they avoided the contraction of at least pneumonic plague by blocking the inhalation of infectious particles. Nonetheless, during the severe plague epidemic in the 1340s, doctors, like the general population, reacted to the disease with fear and horror that led to the neglect of the victims.

A culture of anti-Semitism, unfortunately, coexisted with this developing death culture. As early as 1321 in Languedoc, France, several decades before plague arrived, lepers were accused of contaminating the town's drinking water and were executed. But prior to their end they blamed the Jews for egging them on in this endeavor.[78] However, the lepers faced much discrimination themselves throughout the Middle Ages as they were forced to live separately from the nonleprous population. They were also forced to wear bells around their necks to warn of their approach when they walked through towns. The level of contagion was not high, but lepers' disfiguration from their disease contributed to the fear of and discrimination against them. Leprosy, like plague, has been enveloped by cultural misconceptions of the actual disease. The disease is still commonly referred to as leprosy, even though it was actually renamed Hansen's disease after the nineteenth-century scientist who discovered that it was caused by *Mycobacterium leprae*. The bacterium primarily infects the skin and the mucous membranes. The disease has existed for countless centuries and has proven to be not readily transmissible by touch. Scientists believe a genetic and immune susceptibility account for the acquisition of the bacterium in some people and not in others. It was quite telling that in the midst of the Languedoc lepers' own discrimination, they accused the Jews of assisting them in poisoning the water supply. Of course the lepers did not contaminate the town's water, but they were on the verge of being burnt by the townspeople and they reached out to blame a group of people who were already despised throughout Europe.

An English knight, Sir John Mandeville, wrote a travelogue around this time when the Languedoc lepers accused the Jews of helping them poison the water. Mandeville's work captured some of the most prevalent anti-Semitic sentiments in this century. This knight who supposedly traveled throughout the Far East narrates the customs and mores of the different cultures he encountered in his book. It becomes increasingly evident throughout his narrative that he despises the Jews primarily because of their unwillingness to convert to Christianity whereas he tolerated the Muslims, commonly referred to as Saracens. Muslims believed that Jesus was a prophet and according to Mandeville they potentially could be converted to Christianity. In addition, he claims that Muslims shared this hatred of the Jews because the Koran says the Jews are "wicked and accursed because they will not believe that Jesus was sent from God."[79] Whether or not Mandeville's nonreferenced passage accurately reflects the Koran, he expressed a somewhat popular notion that the Jewish community was *evil* because of its disbelief in the Catholic community's divine being. Instead of trying to understand a much older monotheistic theology, Mandeville labels it evil because it is different from his own.

As Mandeville's narrative progresses, this anti-Semitism deteriorates into paranoia about the Jews destroying the entire Christian community on earth. While traveling near Sumatra, he describes poisonous trees that "the Jews [were] once thought to have poisoned all Christendom [with], as one of them confessed to me; but, blessed be Almighty God, they failed in their purpose."[80] The absurdity of this accusation is all too evident. If the Jews actually procured a poison from this remote tree, how could they poison the entire Christian community around the world? How could they identify and ensure they were only poisoning Christians? Mandeville's attempt to authenticate his account is even more ridiculous: What Jew would confess such a diabolical plot to him? Nonetheless, his idea about Jews attempting to poison Christians paved the way for accusations later in this century that they poisoned wells that caused the plague.

Raymond Crawfurd looks to folklore to explain scapegoating in times of pestilence. In folklore, human as well as animal scapegoats are used to "exorcise pestilence."[81] This folkloric motif of sacrifice can be perceived, for example, in the popular American movie *King Kong*. The natives on the remote island regularly sacrifice a human victim to the huge primate Kong, who is a special type of plague (an affliction), in order to "exorcise" this source of danger from their immediate dwelling. Folktales and folk-like tales actually help us manage our very real values, hopes, and especially fears. For Americans, *King Kong* was not so much about our fear of gigantic gorillas, but perhaps a fear of emerging foreign powers, such as the Soviet Union and Nazi Germany, in 1933 when the original movie was produced. Kong also could be viewed as the fictional embodiment of American anxieties over the pervasive depressed economy that destroyed so many families and communities then. A sacrifice to either menace in both readings of the film might help, or so Americans hoped on some unconscious level, to purge the problem.

But the scapegoating of the Jews in fourteenth-century Europe was "far more deliberate, far more lengthy, far less impassioned than any rite of human sacrifice," as Crawfurd admits.[82] The sacrifice of the Jews was not enacted in a folktale or a movie but by real communities that were terrified of a disease they could not control. Rosemary Horrox explains that this scapegoating met "the familiar human need to find somebody to blame, [and] the accusations may have made the plague seem more manageable, since what man caused could be halted by human efforts."[83] Furthermore, an extreme fear of this disease and the death it caused coupled with a hatred for a group of people who held different beliefs from the predominant Christian community specifically resulted in the Jews being targeted as the human cause of plague. Identification and eradication of this human cause certainly could control the disease. But actually there was no human cause.

The Jews were perhaps also victims of some Christians' projected disdain. As we have seen, many people in the Christian community viewed their own sins, such as pride and greed, as the causes for the divine punishment they suffered in the form of the plague. Some Christians might not have been able to nor wanted to take responsibility for personally inciting their divine being's anger. Others might not have wanted to admit that the Catholic Church's strength was threatened from within its own ranks due to some of the clergy's own corrupt behavior. It may have been easier for these Catholics to project their self-disdain or that held toward their own church onto a different religious group like the Jews. When Jews were falsely accused of poisoning the wells and other sources of water in Savoy, France, in the fall of 1348, the French officials thought the Jews' actions were specifically carried out "in order to destroy and wipe out the entire Christian religion."[84] It was quite telling that fears ran higher among this Catholic community in terms of threats to its own religion than they did regarding the specific threat of plague to all human lives.

Those Christians who hurled these accusations of poisoning against the Jews overlooked the fact that just as many Jews contracted and died from the plague, as Ziegler points out in his history.[85] The accusers did not know yet that a bacterium was responsible for this disease, but their ignorance does not excuse the horrendous discrimination wielded against the Jewish community.

The first accusations regarding the Jews poisoning wells occurred in the south of France in the spring of 1348. By September of this year, several Jews were captured and tortured into giving confessions in Savoy. The Jewish surgeon Balavigny from Villeneuve confessed, along with other Jews, that he received poison from a Jewish boy who had received it from a rabbi along with a letter instructing him to place the poison in public wells. All of the Jews who were forced into these confessions, as well as all of the Jews living in Villeneuve, were "burnt by due legal process" according to the official Savoy document that details these confessions.[86] The persecuting French officials also tortured a few Christians into admitting that they received poison from the Jews. Although this document does not intimate that the tortured Christians sympathized with the accused Jews, we can imagine that they did and that was why they were punished. This document was actually sent as a letter by a French deputy to the citizens of Strasburg in order to justify their acts of murder. In Strasburg, 2,000 Jews were subsequently accused and killed for the same fabricated act of poisoning the wells that spread the plague.[87]

In response to the steadily rising murder of the Jews, Pope Clement VI issued a bull (an official statement of the Catholic Church) to protect the Jews in July 1348. By September he ordered the Catholic clergy to act against anyone who tortured and murdered the Jews. In this rational response to irrational slaughtering, however, the Church's own anti-Semitic position was evident when the pope began his official statement with the caveat: "although we rightly abhor the deceit of the Jews who . . . refuse to . . . accept the Christian faith and salvation."[88] But the pope reminds his see that the Catholic "saviour chose to be born of Jewish stock when he put on mortal flesh" and therefore the Church needs to protect the Jews.[89] The pope also threatened political officials with loss of their offices and, worst of all, excommunication if they killed any Jews. The pope makes it clear in this bull that Christians' sins incited God's anger in the form of plague, and he blatantly dismisses the Jews as the cause of plague as he sees that God has punished them also with this disease.

The pope's order of protection, however, fell on deaf ears. By November 1348 a campaign of massive murder began throughout Germany. Diessenhoven, the German chronicler and a Catholic priest, recorded the persecutions with delight as he tracked them throughout the country. Most gruesome was his report of Jews being immolated in a pit in Horw. Some were half dead and "the stronger of them snatched up cudgels and stones and dashed out the brains of those trying to creep out of the fire."[90] It is hard to imagine that anyone in that pit survived to report the details of this dreadful struggle, and only someone within that pit would have known about it. This chronicler obviously fabricated this event and indulged himself in the Jews' pain and suffering.

Diessenhoven might have experienced disdain toward his own church that he projected onto the Jews. At one point in his account, he praises his divine being "who confounded the ungodly [the Jews] who were plotting the extinction of his church, not realizing that it is founded on a sure rock and who, in trying to overturn it, crushed themselves to death and were damned forever."[91] If this priest was so confident that the Catholic Church had a solid foundation, he might not have had the need to justify that in an account detailing why the Jews deserved to die; instead, he simply would have focused on the Jews' supposed part in spreading the plague. He felt on some level that his church was weakened, and the Jews were a convenient scapegoat for contributing to its cracked foundation. This historian's disdain for the Jewish community is reiterated with the final refrain that this holocaust in Germany was successful and deserved: "And thus, within one year, as I said, all the Jews between Cologne and Austria were burnt—and in Austria they await the same fate, for they are accursed of God."[92]

Yet other rational responses to the plague persisted when some German officials doubted this human cause of plague and did not condone the murder of Jews. A letter sent by Cologne officials to those in Strassburg in January 1349 denounced rumors that the Jews poisoned wells and were responsible for this "unparalleled mortality of Christians."[93] Instead the letter reiterated "divine vengeance and nothing else" as the cause of the plague.[94] Cologne officials urged those in Strassburg to protect the Jews unless proof arose of their guilt. But the murders continued there.

In addition to the 2,000 Jews killed in Strassburg, 12,000 were murdered in Mainz.[95] It is not unreasonable to suggest that the Jews were exterminated in Germany during these plague years on a scale that was duplicated six centuries later by the Nazis. A German Franciscan friar in 1349 revealed in his laconic account of the plague that "throughout Germany, in all but a few places, they were burnt."[96] The Jews who did survive found protection from the King of Aragon and the King of Poland.

Extreme fear of this disease labeled *plague* in conjunction with a predominant culture's discrimination against a different group of people resulted in human targets of blame. Proposed human sources of plague produced far more sinister consequences than proposed divine and even astrological ones. When the Christian community blamed its own followers for this form of divine punishment in fourteenth-century Europe, the solution for plague was to rectify their own behavior. Planetary causes simply were felt to be beyond their control. But when a politically powerful segment of the Catholic community offered the Jews as the cause of plague, the solution was extermination.

Extreme emotional reactions to plague along with proposed divine and human causes persist in subsequent centuries when the disease reemerges. And even after the bacterial cause of so-called plague is discovered near the end of the nineteenth century, plague maintains its power to induce irrationality and discrimination.

CHAPTER 4

Fifteenth- through Seventeenth-Century Europe

We had a routine. Every night when I awakened Lenny for his 4 A.M. AZT, I would shake his left shoulder and quickly jump back from his bed. He always woke up swinging while assuming the shooting position. Then he would ask, "Did I get you?" Lenny served as a marine in Vietnam during the early 1970s. He was not so sure if his platoon was in Cambodia fighting, but he was positive that he acquired his powerful addiction to heroin during those countless nights of deafening gunfire, unbearable levels of humidity accompanied by relentless insects, and a palpable hunger to survive. The heroin enabled him to survive by deadening the shock of this reality.

When Lenny was honorably discharged from his duty in 1973, he left behind his devoted service to our country—after all he never missed his mark—and the high levels of adrenaline produced daily from the constant assault on his own mortality, but he could not leave the heroin. Lenny had no problem holding good construction jobs when he returned to New York, thanks to his work ethic—he never missed a day of work until I met him in 1989—and his strong frame.

When he met Anna shortly after he returned home, she fell in love with his strength and his duty to work and, of course, to her. He was also rather kind. For more than 15 years of their marriage, he protected her from knowing about his after-work crawls to the flophouses where he procured the drug he had grown to rely on for survival in Vietnam. He also inadvertently protected her from the virus he had eventually picked up from sharing the instrument of his heroin delivery with others, which he revealed to me one night after I knew him about a year. He explained that if he had not used condoms, he would have passed his addiction to Anna and their unborn offspring. This protective behavior also explained why they did not have children in spite of their culture urging them otherwise. Anna did not speak much English. She primarily spoke the Spanish of her native Puerto Rico, as Lenny did, but he spoke fluent English in part because he relished acting as her personal translator, especially when she spent long hours with him during his increasingly regular hospitalizations.

In 1989 when Lenny still needed time to digest his AIDS diagnosis, I understood why he did not discuss it with Anna. He felt ashamed, and he was proud to be a good husband and provider. Admission of his drug use, he thought, would have diminished his stature in Anna's eyes. He did not appear to be endangering her health because he used precautions during sexual intercourse, so I did not press the issue so much then. But three years later when Lenny was still living with AIDS, a somewhat amazing feat in 1992, I was perplexed and a bit more concerned that his revelation to her was not forthcoming.

During the winter of 1992, Lenny was admitted with his seventh or eighth bout of PCP. By now his brawny physique had deflated into an emaciated figure, the common face of AIDS then. He was in the final stage of his disease. He had not worked in months, he could barely walk to the bathroom from his hospital bed, and his appetite had fled. By this time, I had grown fairly close with Anna also, and we always managed to communicate with each other about Lenny's eating, sleeping, and toileting routines in spite of our language barrier.

Shortly before he died during that winter, I asked Lenny again if he had told Anna the truth about his illness. I thought that even though they practiced safe sex, she should still be tested in case one of those condoms was faulty, and his revelation would have helped her understand his devolution into a bedridden shadow. Lenny said he did not have the courage to tell her. "Why not?" I asked. "She loves you so much, Lenny." He sadly retorted, "What would she think of me, Gina?"

"What will they think?" This common refrain has been spoken by many other AIDS sufferers and serves as their explanation for why they did not reveal their disease to families, friends, lovers, acquaintances, and employers. They were terrified of the judgment. So were people in London during the 1665 plague outbreak there. They feared infamy and, worst of all, quarantine for carrying a disease viewed as plague.

Plague nestled into endemic status in European countries and recurred approximately every 5–12 years after the 1348 catastrophe produced devastating losses there. Those mortality rates were not reached again until the 1665 epidemic in London, but milder outbreaks occurred in European countries in these interim centuries. For example, the 1471 plague in England, probably one of the worst of this period, killed 10–15 percent of the population there within four months.[1]

Fourteenth-century perceptions of plague persisted during the fifteenth and sixteenth centuries; however, fewer writings were produced on the subject. One example was John Lydgate's poem written in the first half of the fifteenth century in England. "A Dietary, and a Doctrine for Pestilence" provided advice on avoiding the plague and was widely circulated. In the first three stanzas, the poet advises his readers to avoid "the stroke of pestilence" by staying away from "infected places" and especially by avoiding the "black mist," the refrain of this section.[2] Pestilence was still a popular epithet for the disease. Also presenting it as a "stroke" suggests that some divine being is wielding an instrument of punishment at human subjects. Yet Lydgate actually favors the more ecological cause of the disease: miasma ("black mist").

Ecological causes of the plague grant humans a little more control in preventing the disease, and the majority of Lydgate's poem is devoted to dietary preventives for the plague that involve more than food. He advocates the Aristotelian path of moderation by discouraging too much work, too much sleep, and gluttony in general. But he places the greatest stock in sensible eating.

Lydgate's more sanguine approach to the plague—he believes it can be avoided by following his instructions—may be attributed to the fact that he did not witness massive suffering and death from the disease. Preventing the disease seems to have been more within human control during these less virulent outbreaks. But Lydgate's writing does not escape the culture of death that emerged with the fourteenth-century epidemic. Toward the end of his poem, he captures the transient pleasures of life with death hovering near: "No worldly joy lasts here but awhile."[3]

Several fifteenth-century paintings explore death. With minor outbreaks of the plague in the fifteenth century, survival was a reality and this may be why we see the fear of death sometimes depicted along with the hope of living. A portrait from England in this period, "The Three Living and the Three Dead," shows three royal men, one of whom is a bishop, standing face to face with three skeletons staring intently at them while they pray. The three skeletons mirror the three mortal men, especially as the skeleton matched with the bishop wears a miter. This portrait depicts life and death at a standoff with the winner undecided.[4]

Another late fifteenth-century painting from France, "The Physician and Death," presents the popular image of a physician examining urine in a large glass vial.[5] Uroscopy was a common method of diagnosing disorders that stemmed from an imbalance in the body's humors. In this period, a popular medical theory of disease causality was that the proper balance of yellow bile, black bile, phlegm, and blood produced good health, and any imbalance in one or more of these humors produced disease. In this painting, as the ornately clad physician attempts to make his diagnosis by peering at the vial of urine he holds up, a draped skeleton enters and touches his robe. The doctor is reminded at this moment that diagnosing any disease is ultimately futile with surprise visits from death.

In these two paintings, the living survive, but other works of art during the fifteenth to sixteenth centuries deal with the absolute triumph of death. The narrator of the anonymous poem "Disputation between the Body and Worms" visits a tomb in a church during a powerful plague outbreak.[6] The narrator dreams about a discussion between the supposedly rotting female corpse in the tomb and the worms who greedily feed on her body. She pleads with the insects to abandon her beautiful body but to no avail. The worms believe they are doing her a favor since no one else will assist in decomposing her corpse. These minions of death grant no allowances to the pleading woman whose earthly beauty is quickly fading.

The famous sixteenth-century Flemish painting "The Triumph of Death" by Pieter Bruegel the Elder perhaps embodies the tyranny of death most poignantly.[7] In this painting, we enter a hopeless war scene between skeletons and humans. The army of skeletons has just arrived by sea to mercilessly plunder everyone they find alive in a village. The skeletons are gleeful in their work. As in Petrarch's fourteenth-century poem with the same title, death pervades every niche of the canvas.

Art immersed in the death culture of this period certainly expressed the cultural fear of death; one could say that death was depicted so often in an effort to control it or at least to come to terms with it. Unfortunately, this fear of death continued to take the form of scapegoating, albeit on a more minor scale in comparison to the fourteenth century. In 1494, *The Nuremberg Chronicle* recorded that all beggars were exiled from Nuremberg in Germany because they were deemed to be plague carriers.[8] And in Lyons, France, in 1565, the town magistrates were advised by a physician to closely watch criminals "who grease and smear the walls and doors of rich houses with matter from buboes."[9] Marginal groups continued to be a target for the societal convergence of fears about plague.

At the turn of the sixteenth to the seventeenth century in London, a self-proclaimed physician named Simon Forman wrote two plague treatises that provide further insight into perceptions of the disease during less deadly occurrences. According to Barbara Howard Traister, whose book collects many of Forman's writings from manuscripts found only in British libraries, Forman suffered and recovered from the plague during the 1592 outbreak in

London.[10] His illness provoked him to write a plague treatise the following year that opined two medieval causes for the disease: astrological and divine. In this treatise, Forman distinguishes between different types of buboes or "sores" that originate from planetary influences.[11] Buboes caused by Mars were very painful, quick to erupt, and more infectious than those caused by Saturn.

On the other hand, black areas of discoloration on the skin's surface had a divine origin, when in reality this discoloration resulted from the lack of oxygen to the skin usually produced by septicemic plague. Forman called them "God's tokens," and he thought they were a result of society's ills, which included corrupt clergy, greedy merchants and landlords, and unvirtuous women who "wore ridiculous clothes."[12] This is not the first time we have seen these behaviors offered as causes of divine punishment in the form of plague.

Forman's second treatise on plague, written in 1607, focused on more "practical" interventions for treating the disease.[13] For example, he detailed how to lance buboes and apply salve to assist in the healing process. He also offered a warm environment and avoidance of onions as part of his "dietary" for the plague. Forman shared Lydgate's view that the plague could be prevented and even treated, especially since he actually recovered from the disease a few years earlier.

Even though the prevalent medieval view of divine causality persisted into the seventeenth century, Lydgate and Forman moved toward more practical interventions for contending with the disease. This shift signified a more scientific response to the plague that continued during the 1665 London epidemic.

This next epidemic in England actually began a few years earlier on the Asian continent, and then extended into Italy, Germany, France, and Spain. Amsterdam was hit hard in 1663 just as England was gearing up for a war with Holland, its trading partner and rival. Although war between the two countries was not officially declared until February 1665, fear of the Dutch carrying the plague on to British shores was intense. Ships arriving from Amsterdam were quarantined for 30 days on the River Thames ever since 1663.

The first case of the official last severe outbreak during the second global plague pandemic (1346–1722) was declared by a London searcher.[14] Searchers were older women hired by local parishes to determine causes of death. This case was determined on Christmas Eve of 1664 outside the walls of London in St. Giles in the Fields. As the number of cases grew throughout 1665, 40 percent of the population left London, including King Charles II and his court. The plague traveled to the countryside with those who fled and killed 100,000 there. Of the 300,000 people left in London, 100,000 died. The mortality rate of this epidemic approached 18 percent until it finally calmed down by the summer of 1666.[15]

The circulation of the weekly *Bill of Mortality* in London—in a way, a precursor of today's *Morbidity and Mortality Weekly Report* produced by the Centers for Disease Control—concretized the reality of daily suffering by recording the number of weekly burials and causes of death, alongside a more pleasant splattering of the numbers of marriages and christenings. Sometimes, however, the *Bill*'s veracity in recording plague as a cause of death was questionable. Several Londoners were not completely honest about plague killing their family members because of the discrimination that typically surrounded the plague victim.

Writings from the seventeenth to eighteenth centuries that mention the 1665 London plague reveal, however, more of a transition toward scientific perceptions and reactions to plague. Samuel Pepys' *Diary* devotes a couple of hundred pages to the eruption, progression, and departure of the plague in London.[16] John Dryden's heroic poem "Annus Mirabilis," written during 1666 to praise England's virtue in war with the Dutch, briefly mentions the plague.[17] And Daniel Defoe's *A Journal of the Plague Year* remains one of the most popular references today for the 1665 London epidemic, even though it is narrated by the fictional H.F. and was written in Marseilles, France, 57 years after the London outbreak.[18] Defoe's work best captures both older and emerging views of plague.

During this time, the disease still retained the label of *plague*. Pepys called it "plague" one month after he noted its arrival in London.[19] Defoe's narrator calls it "pestilence" and when describing Londoners' extreme reactions to the disease, such as suicide, it is a "scourge."[20] Yet new labels for the disease appeared, such as "visitation." This label actually suggests that there is hope for the disease's departure if it has just dropped in for a "visit." Defoe seemed particularly hopeful about the plague's permanent departure from London when he wrote his journal in 1722, given that the last part of his long subtitle is "the last great visitation in 1665."[21] His subtitle seems to will the disease's absence from England, and the 1665 epidemic indeed was the last "great visitation" there.

Divine attributions for plague in 1665 persisted but need to be understood within the political atmosphere of this period. The nonroyal military leader Oliver Cromwell rose to power in England throughout the 1640s, which ultimately resulted in the beheading of the Catholic king, Charles I, in 1649. Cromwell's rule is considered the Interregnum period in English history. In broad terms, during this time the country was divided between supporters of the monarchy and supporters of Cromwell. The monarchy's supporters tended to hold on to traditional Catholic beliefs and practices, while Cromwell's rule facilitated and favored Protestant sects, especially Puritans, many of whom had already settled on American shores. By 1660, Charles II, who had been in exile during Cromwell's rule, restored royal power along with tolerance for Catholics.

A popular belief at that time was that this civil war was particularly sinful and incurred plague. Defoe's narrator is outspoken about the role of the restored monarchy in this plague outbreak. When H.F. describes King Charles II's departure from London in June 1665 as the plague cases begin to rise, he claims "their crying Vices" were responsible for "bringing that terrible Judgment upon the whole Nation."[22] He simply could be criticizing the monarchy's flight from the city, but it seems like this admonishment extends to their political actions during the restoration of their rule. Nonetheless, the monarchy is assumed to be responsible for God's judgment in the form of plague.

According to the Mootes, many people regardless of religious alliances continued to believe that "God alone brought the plague as a judgment on a sinning people."[23] In his *Diary,* Pepys did not attribute blame to any religious or political group for plague's arrival, but at moments he sees a divine role in the disease's spread. For example, Pepys' fears about the plague's prevalence in October 1665 are buttressed by his hopes that "God send a decrease" in the number of deaths.[24] For Pepys, if a divine source was not explicitly responsible for plague's appearance, it may have been capable of making the disease disappear.

Astrologic causes for plague also persisted in this period. The Mootes discuss the conjoining of Saturn and Jupiter in 1663, a planetary alignment with great portent for the fourteenth-century epidemic, and Saturn appeared to approach Mars in November 1664. Astrologers were quite popular in the 1660s and viewed these events as indicators of plague's arrival in December 1664. In addition, on Christmas Eve of this year, as the first plague case was being determined, a comet appeared in the sky that astrologers and many other people saw as a sure sign of plague's arrival. Another comet sighting occurred in March 1665 and the plague cases kept coming.[25] A famous member of the recently formed Royal Society in 1662, Edmund Halley, observed these two comets.

John Dryden devoted a few stanzas of his 1666 poem "Annus Mirabilis" to astrologic causes of this plague. His poem, unlike Defoe's *Journal,* sympathizes with the restored monarchy. Dryden has the king speak near the end about how the Great Fire of London in September 1666 was a punishment for the country's sin of civil war.[26] When the city then speaks to the king in the poem, the comets of 1664 and 1665 are viewed as direct causes of both plague and fire: " . . . two dire comets which have scourg'd the town/In their own plague and fire . . . ."[27] Dryden uses divine vengeance discourse that usually surrounds plague without specifically mentioning a divine source. The comets themselves "scourge" London with plague and fire because of the country's long division before the restoration of Charles II.

Defoe saw the astrologic significance of the comets, but ultimately assigned them a divine source. H.F. describes the "stars" that appeared before plague and the fire as "the Forerunners and Warnings of God's Judgments."[28] The comets were not the direct cause of the plague as they were in Dryden, but they were the sign of imminent divine punishment.

Climatic causes of plague persisted from the medieval period during the London epidemic. The apothecary William Boghurst proposed that people who did not live their lives with moderation, Lydgate's advice two centuries before him, were prone to contract the plague from miasma, or bad air.[29] Pepys saw a direct correlation between the outside temperature and the number of plague cases. Toward the end of December 1665, he recorded, "the weather hath been frosty these eight or nine days, and so we hope for an abatement of the plague the next week."[30] Pepys was unwittingly prescient in his observation that warmer weather results in more plague cases. The cold weather provokes *Xenopsylla cheopis*, the flea that carries *Yersinia pestis*, to hibernate and it does not transmit the bacterium outside of the ideal temperature range of 13–34 degrees Celsius, or 55–93 degrees Fahrenheit.[31] Pepys' observation looks forward to more biological explanations for the disease.

Only a few years before this plague time, Charles II chartered the Royal Society, one of the first organizations in Europe devoted to producing new knowledge in the natural sciences. Well-known members of the Society included Sir Isaac Newton, who theorized the laws of gravity; Robert Boyle, who theorized the laws of gases; and Robert Hooke, who wrote the first collection of observations through a microscope. These discoveries show a society that was no longer solely seeking for answers in the divine realm. By 1665, the age of humanism was well underway. People now believed in their own inherent ability to discover and solve problems in their environment.

In this milieu, we should not be surprised to see scientific causes proposed for this disease. The apothecary Boghurst saw value in a new Italian disease causality theory: *seminaria*. The Italians studied syphilis and proposed that "atomlike seedlets" carried the disease, and Boghurst applied this theory to plague.[32] Similarly, Boghurst thought that plague *seminaria* existed but were not visible to the naked eye; however, they were responsible for producing the effects of the disease in humans that everyone did see. These theories illustrated a rudimentary germ theory of disease.

By the time Defoe wrote his *Journal* in the early eighteenth century, divine causes of plague were still being weighed alongside more scientific ones. Early on H.F. has a philosophical discussion with his brother about his decision to flee London as the number of plague cases rises daily. But H.F. believes that it might be "the Will of Heaven" for him to stay in the city and, if that is the case, God will "preserve me in the midst of all Death and Danger that would surround me."[33] Conversely, if he leaves, God will punish him with plague, or so he thinks. H.F.'s brother, a merchant, points out a flaw in this line of thinking by mentioning Muslims he met abroad on business who believed they were "predestined" by God to *not* contract plague.[34] With this sense of self-protection, they mingled with infected people and consequently died. His brother's point is that there is no guarantee of God's protection from plague.

The questioning attitude of H.F.'s brother and the mounting dead bodies observed throughout the city by Defoe's narrator lead him to contemplate more scientific causes of the disease. As H.F. discusses his objections to the practice of quarantining, he proposes that "the Calamity was spread by Infection, that is to say, by some certain Steams, or Fumes, which the Physicians call *Effluvia*."[35] Richard Bradley, a physician contemporary of Defoe, called the medium of plague infection *effluvia* that carried insects floating through the air, which in turn could enter the stomachs of animals and kill them.[36] The *effluvia* may resemble the older notion of a miasma, but the insects within it resemble the *seminaria* of the Italians and Boghurst.

Any infectious disease has a reservoir, or domain where it lives, and it can be transmitted by air, insect bites, exchange of bodily fluids, or touch, for example, to a vulnerable host who can further transmit it to another one. Medicine today focuses on breaking the chain of infection in order to stop its spread. People in the seventeenth and eighteenth centuries had a dim sense of this chain of infection when they stayed away from people with active plague, like Boghurst did in his practice as an apothecary.[37] Pepys also intuits that escape from sick people will prevent contraction of the disease. One night Pepys' coachman falls suddenly ill and Pepys quickly departs the coach to find another one. One month later, his servant lies down on his bed complaining of a headache and Pepys hurries about to have him removed from his home.[38] Furthermore, Defoe's narrator recognizes that silent carriers of plague "breathed Death in every Place, and upon every Body who came near them," and that no one contracts the disease unless contact with the infected has occurred.[39]

Defoe's work, however, does not wholeheartedly embrace these newer theories about plague's causality. For instance, H.F. may endorse *effluvia* as a cause of plague, but he later denies the existence of microscopes that could potentially identify the bugs. H.F. will not allow that organisms, which he calls "living Creatures," can be seen through a microscope and he bolsters his claim by lying, "we had no Microscopes at that Time."[40] Defoe certainly must have known there were microscopes in 1665. Robert Hooke's *Microscopy* was published in the beginning of 1665 and Pepys bought a copy of it. Furthermore, Pepys enthusiastically mentioned the microscope that he and his dinner guests look through after a dinner party in his home.[41] H.F.'s denial of the microscope's existence captured the opinion of those people who did not want to grant nondivine causes of plague. Even though H.F. continues to employ more scientific terms for the disease such as "contagion," he thought that divine intervention was ultimately responsible for plague's disappearance: "Nothing, but the immediate Finger of God, nothing, but omnipotent Power could have done it."[42] These divine causality theories must have provided security for Defoe's readers who were not comfortable with emerging scientific theories.

Traditional reactions to plague persisted from the medieval period during this time. The disease's toll on London's population was grim, and so it is not surprising that people continued to react with fear. During the week of September 12–19, 1665, 7,165 people died from the plague with nightly burials in the 1,000–2,000 range.[43] Even Pepys, who always stayed focused on his successes at the Exchequer, could not shake his fear during this month. Although he has his health and financial security, he is consumed with "the consideration of the sickliness of the season during this great plague [which] mortif[ies] me."[44]

Even before this tragic week in September, fear took the form of flight, especially for those who had the financial means. In the spring of 1665, as the number of deaths and quarantines steadily rose, the well-to-do peers and gentry retreated to their country homes while leaving their servants behind. By the end of this summer, 200,000 people had left London, including the king and his court.[45] And when Defoe's narrator presents the statistics from the weekly *Bills of Mortality* in September 1665, he proclaims that "the best Physick against the Plague is to run away from it."[46] Plague-ridden London, however, remained home to nonroyal city and government officials; business owners; servants and laborers; and those directly serving plague patients such as nurses, doctors, pharmacists, searchers, and watchers (men placed in front of quarantined homes to "watch" that no one left or entered).

Reactions of despair and hedonism also persisted during the 1665 epidemic. Although Pepys generally remained sanguine about plague's departure, he became inured to the sight of dead bodies, which could be considered a form of despair. When he talks with an associate in the road in early October 1665, he notes "the bearers with a dead corps[e] of the plague" pass by, and then reflects "but Lord, to see what custom is, that I am come almost to think nothing of it."[47] Defoe captures despair in his vignettes of several Londoners, but one portrait is particularly memorable: A man is so burdened with sorrow from the death of his family that his head slowly sinks down between his shoulders, where it remains for one year before his own death from this physical impossibility.[48]

On the other hand, hedonism was prevalent in the town of Colchester, a few hours ride from London. Plague visited there from August 1665 to December 1666, resulting in a 40–50 percent population loss. It is no wonder that many people in the Dutch-settled section of Colchester engaged in "lusty singing and carousing in taverns long after the nighttime curfew."[49] These indulgences must have served as a Band-Aid for witnessing such fatalities.

Defoe also highlights hedonistic behavior back in London. Rowdy tavern goers sit by the tavern window every night and mock the death carts that pass by on their way to the pits. H.F. is most offended by their taunting of a man whom he has befriended in his despair over the loss of his wife and children. When H.F. attempts to explain to the revelers that the plague is no laughing matter, especially since it is divine judgment, they mock him. H.F. happily reports that their hedonistic responses to plague were punished by God, as each of them dies from the disease.[50]

But newer reactions to plague emerged at this time and were influenced by this general turn away from the heavens in search of causes for the disease. To a large degree, public health sanitary measures stemmed from a growing sense of communicable transmission. In May 1665, the mayor of London ordered all owners of shops and homes to clean the street in front of their residences daily.[51] Realistically, none of the three forms of plague would have been prevented with this cleaning, but the mayor's order constituted a public health measure to prevent person-to-person transmission of the disease. The city also ordered the killing of all dogs and cats in June of this year because both animals were thought to be disease vectors.[52] Identification of the rat in the chain of plague infection would have to wait two more centuries. In addition, more personal sanitary measures were witnessed in the practice of butchers placing money in vinegar during transactions with customers and by a drastic change in the fashion of wearing periwigs.[53] Pepys commented that people stopped buying them because they feared the hair was procured from dead plague victims and they did not want to contract the disease.[54]

Quarantining was a widely instituted public health sanitary measure, although 1665 was not the first time it was implemented. During the mid-fourteenth-century plague in Aragon, the king there ordered high volume areas of plague to be quarantined. The plague of 1423 in Venice inspired quarantine in the form of the first plague hospital or "lazaretto." And Defoe discusses King James I's 1603 quarantine act in London, which was based on an earlier one issued in 1583.[55]

Quarantining in 1665 London, however, happened on a larger scale because of the sheer number of people infected with the disease. After the first plague deaths were made public on April 27, 1665, King Charles II issued the order for quarantine: For 40 days from the time of the last plague death in the house, everyone would be contained therein whether or not they were sick.[56] Pepys was distraught to see the first quarantined homes in Drury Lane "with a red cross upon the doors, and 'Lord have mercy upon us' " written upon them, the visible refrain for all of these homes.[57]

Perhaps the greater than 7,000 deaths during the week of September 12–19, 1665 would have numbered more than 10,000 if not for the quarantined homes the uninfected encountered throughout London. Nonetheless, this act of widespread quarantining signified a change in medieval reactions to the disease. Londoners may have attended church services up to twice daily during this time,[58] but their sole focus was shifting away from rectifying sins in order to halt the disease and more toward sanitary measures for accomplishing this goal.

The widely instituted quarantine throughout London, however, did produce its own set of reactions. Defoe was the most critical of this public health measure in his *Journal*, and even places H.F. in the objectionable position of a city-appointed "examiner."[59] Examiners searched for potential plague patients and gave the order to quarantine the homes when they found them. Watchmen were posted outside quarantined homes in order to keep any potential escapees inside. H.F. discusses the "violence" often wielded against these watchers as family members were desperate to escape.[60] As a matter of fact, Defoe has H.F. argue that the very act of quarantining induces a desire for flight that otherwise would not have occurred.

Quarantining also provoked deceit about the disease. Defoe shows us families who paid their parish officers to lie in their recording of the cause of death when it was plague. These payoffs affected the accuracy of the number of plague deaths presented in the *Bills of Mortality*. This false reporting, however, "spare[d] people the ignominy of plague in their family or neighborhood."[61] Although we have been witnessing more scientific responses to plague during this epidemic, people certainly remained terrified of the disease itself and the judgment that often accompanied it.

Accusations of deception were cast against nurses who were appointed to quarantined homes. They were sealed inside the home with the sick victim and family, and often they died along with other healthy family members. Many Londoners thought that nurses covered warm corpses with blankets in order to stop the buboes from erupting.[62] And Defoe discusses rumors of nurses who apparently murdered their patients in order to shorten the length of the quarantine. Defoe actually denounces these rumors, but they serve as more fodder to support his argument against quarantining.[63] If the quarantined patient was determined to have died from a disease other than plague, the house would not be isolated for another 40 days.

The widespread practice of quarantining in 1665 London constituted a quite different response to plague in comparison to the medieval world. Scapegoating also had a different flavor in 1665. For instance, the Jews "were not scapegoats" during this plague outbreak.[64] But the Jewish community was only a couple hundred strong in London because they had been expelled from England in 1290 under Edward I and only recently permitted to return from abroad under Cromwell in 1656. They might not have been targets of blame in 1665 because their presence was not as prevalent as it was in other fourteenth-century European countries.

No blatant discriminatory actions were wielded against the poor either, but they served as convenient targets of blame for plague's existence by the wealthier classes. The Mootes explain that "rich and middle-income Londoners believed that the 'sluttishness' of the poor and their overcrowded housing, called 'pestered places,' bred disease."[65] In this view, the poor were "immoral," one meaning of "sluttish" at this time,[66] by virtue of their socio-economic class, and this "immorality" caused plague. During the next plague pandemic, the Chinese people in Hong Kong and the United States are blamed more blatantly for causing plague for similar reasons as the poor were in 1665 London.

CHAPTER 5

The Nineteenth through Twentieth Centuries

The third and last plague pandemic to date began by the end of the nineteenth century and ceased by the mid-twentieth century, thanks to the discovery and effectiveness of several antibiotics, such as streptomycin.[1] In his recent history of the third pandemic, Myron Echenberg proposes that "at least 15 million" people died worldwide.[2] Population losses, however, were not as concentrated in any one country during this visit of plague, perhaps because of the ability of humans to now travel more globally and take the disease with them.

This pandemic emerged in China in 1855. By the time it left that country one century later, 2 million people were dead.[3] From China, the plague traveled to Hong Kong, where the first case was diagnosed in May 1894.[4] In August 1896, Bombay was hit and the disease did not leave India until the 1920s with the death toll at 12 million.[5] By 1900, New Zealand, Australia, Alexandria, Portugal, Africa, South America, Hawaii, and California were visited by plague. I focus primarily on Hong Kong, where the bacterial cause of the disease was discovered, and on California, where the disease touched down on American shores for the first time. Both locations share very similar cultural perceptions of the disease.

For the first time in its history, Hong Kong was hit hard by plague. Within six months of the first diagnosed case in May 1894, the number of infected rose to 2,679, with 2,552 deaths in a total population of 246,000.[6] Although only 1 percent of the Hong Kong population perished from the disease, it devastated the city and produced reactions reminiscent of those of earlier centuries.

Gone were the days when planetary misalignments and comets were proposed as causes of the disease; however, divine explanations persisted in 1894. The white European population in Hong Kong, namely the British, had occupied the country for quite a few decades. Although they only experienced a few cases of plague (11 out of 4,000, to be exact) due in part to their remoteness from rat-infested close living quarters where the Chinese lived,[7] the Chinese considered them as recipients of divine punishment. Hostility toward the colonizers certainly existed. The Chinese felt that a railroad line constructed by the British was built on Chinese babies and the gods punished everyone with plague, regardless of race. Even Buddhist nuns in China viewed a global immorality, regardless of ethnicity, as provocation for the gods' punishment with plague in China.[8]

Fear and denial remained familiar reactions to plague in 1894 Hong Kong. With so many deaths occurring rapidly in such a short period of time, fear of contracting the disease provoked many to leave. A little more than a month after the epidemic emerged in Hong Kong, 80,000 Chinese retreated to the mainland.[9] A fear of admitting the disease's presence in Hong Kong resulted in falsifying reports like we saw in 1665 London. The registrar of deaths denied plague even after the first 40 cases in May, according to a Hong Kong newspaper. The registrar reported these deaths that occurred in the most affected urban district as bowel and lung ailments.[10]

Plague, however, could not be denied, especially as the cases mounted, and two prominent scientists arrived in Hong Kong to find the cause of the disease. Within a month of the first diagnosed case, the Japanese scientist Shibasaburo Kitasato, who trained under Robert Koch in Germany, and the French scientist Alexandre Yersin, who trained at the Pasteur Institute in Paris, arrived to begin their work of deriving specimens from dead victims. Kitasato claimed the discovery of the bacterium from the first autopsy he performed. He drew blood from the corpse and injected it into mice in which he detected the same bacillus. Yersin also was busily searching to identify the organism during the autopsies he performed. He was not convinced that Kitasato found the plague bacillus because he could not readily isolate it in the blood of patients at the time of their deaths. Yersin detected another bacillus in the buboes of these patients that turned out to be the one that caused the disease. Yet, Yersin did not receive the recognition he deserved until 1954, when the bacillus was renamed *Yersinia pestis*.[11]

Dr. James Lowson, a British doctor in Hong Kong who happened to diagnose the first case there, favored Kitasato and reported his findings to the prominent British medical journal *Lancet* near the end of June 1894, while Yersin's results were not published in the same journal until August. *Lancet* still referred to the disease as *plague* in spite of imminent confirmation of a microbial cause of the disease; as a matter of fact, the medical journal called it "oriental plague."[12] Plague now acquired an ethnic identifier.

This newly acquired ethnic quality of the disease was perhaps influenced by the ruling white British colonists' disdain of their own failure to stop the disease's return in one of their colonies. This disdain was projected onto the Chinese, the ethnic group that was the most affected by plague in Hong Kong. Projected disdain as a reaction to plague would be expected from Victorian England because of the country's many successes in this period. This era was eponymously named after Queen Victoria of England who prided her long reign on emblematizing the values of her nineteenth-century British subjects. The British principally valued the notion of *progress,* which they achieved on a national and international scale. For example, England benefited from the age of industrialization as railroads were built around the country, which assisted in the trade of new goods such as coal and steel. Overall, industrialization raised the standard of living for the middle and wealthier classes, while poverty continued to be a reality for the working classes.

The English nation in the nineteenth century also annexed Charles Dickens, the Bronte sisters, and George Eliot to their pantheon of great authors. The British scientific academy, which could boast Sir Isaac Newton and Robert Boyle as former members, welcomed Charles Darwin and his theory of evolution based on natural selection. And internationally, England could glory in the extension of her rule to countries all over the globe, including most of Canada; several islands off of the United States coast; and parts of Africa, Australia, New Zealand, India, and Hong Kong.

England's domestic and international successes made it difficult for its subjects to readily accept the return of the nasty little disease that seemed so *medieval.* As John Kelly aptly puts it in his history on plague, the disease's return "in late nineteenth-century China horrified the self-confident Victorians."[13] The Victorian ethos of progress was halted by plague's reappearance. A scapegoat certainly would assist in easing British anxieties over any diminishment in their own sense of progress.

The Chinese in Hong Kong were viewed as "immoral" by the British, and this immorality bred the disease of plague in the British mind. Edward Marriott points out that because plague did not affect the European population like it affected the Chinese, this was "clear testimony [for the British] to the causal link between moral decay and disease."[14] In reality, the close living quarters of Chinese in Hong Kong enabled the rats to scurry between homes, carrying their infected fleas, thus accounting for the increased numbers of Chinese, as opposed to British, infected with the disease.

Plague as a result of immorality was not a foreign concept to the British, if we recall. The medieval English view was that sins incurred God's wrath in the form of plague. Now in the nineteenth-century British colony of Hong Kong, the British specifically assigned immorality to the Chinese because they were ethnically and culturally different. Immorality for the British became an ethnic flaw. The Chinese were immoral *because* they were not British. Hong Kong might have been *subsumed* under the British Empire, but the Hong Kong residents were not *assumed* to be British. Plague within this progressive empire needed to be explained, and if Chinese immorality was offered as the cause of plague's return, British success would not be diminished in their minds.

The ruling ethnic and social group in Hong Kong found a human cause for plague in spite of the fact that Kitasato and Yersin were there in the process of discovering the bacteriological one. This British scapegoating was most evident in their quarantining policy. Quickly after the first case of plague was diagnosed by Dr. Lowson in May 1894, a makeshift plague ship hospital named *Hygeia* was created on the Hong Kong waterfront. However, it only admitted Chinese patients. Furthermore, Chinese patients were no longer permitted to visit their community hospital in the city. Dr. Lowson thought "it would be impossible to prevent contagion spreading into the community" if the Chinese continued to visit their community hospital.[15] Of course if they had been allowed quarantine in the community hospital, plague prevention would have been possible. The ship hospital quarantine was for the benefit of the British, not the Chinese. Keeping as many plague-ridden Chinese offshore dimmed the plague's presence in the eyes of the colonial government.

The Chinese, however, did not readily succumb to these quarantine orders to board the ship hospital, and they even raised questions about the British government's motives in placing them there. Were they to be the objects of scientific experiments? Subsequently, the British government ended the quarantine orders for the *Hygeia*, and instead turned a deplorable glass factory, in close proximity to the plague pits, where the dead bodies were buried, into a new hospital for the Chinese. On the other hand, a police station in the same district of Hong Kong was converted into a plague hospital for the few Europeans who contracted the disease; apparently, a land-based hospital for Europeans could not spread the disease. Also, the European hospital provided beds, food, and nursing care, unlike the glass factory hospital where Chinese patients slept on the floor.[16]

A few years later, discrimination against the Chinese continued in San Francisco, California, when plague arrived on American shores for the first time. Plague was supposedly introduced to the port city by a Japanese or Australian ship that unwittingly carried the rats and infected humans.[17] The first case of the disease was diagnosed in early March 1900 in a Chinese man who lived in Chinatown. Immediately after a white doctor examined the patient, the discrimination began. A quarantine was ordered by the city for

Chinatown, which was cordoned off with ropes. Two months later, with nine deaths from plague, a federal response ensued that again focused solely on the Chinese. The surgeon general ordered another quarantine for Chinatown, as well as mandatory vaccines for its residents. By1900, Dr. Yersin had created a plague antiserum to be administered after infection with the bacterium, and the Russian scientist Waldemer Haffkine developed an experimental, preventive vaccine. The possible removal of all Chinese to Angel Island off of San Francisco also was proposed by officials.

A few Chinese consented to the vaccine, mass vaccination did not occur, and the Chinese population never was removed to Angel Island. The quarantine of Chinatown was actually lifted by a rational judge in mid-June 1900. He said the order had been "discriminating in its character."[18] Indeed, the discriminatory nature of the quarantine was highlighted when a Chinese grocer in Chinatown filed a lawsuit with the city because the white plumber and coal dealer next to his store were not quarantined.

But the discrimination against the Chinese did not cease. President Theodore Roosevelt delivered a speech near the end of 1901 that reinforced the Chinese Exclusion Act of 1882. This law attempted to limit any more Chinese immigration into the United States and to prevent what was popularly referred to as *coolie* labor. This slang term for Chinese laborers, which has its origins in an Indian Hindu tribe, was applied to any unskilled laborer. White Americans were threatened economically by Chinese laborers who would work for lower wages, and by Chinese success in the mining industry and in urban businesses after their emigration to America throughout the nineteenth century. The outbreak of plague in Chinatown was a perfect excuse for Roosevelt's reenactment of this inherently discriminatory 1882 law. By this time, the Chinese were no longer perceived as just an economic threat to the white community but as a medical one, as well. Limiting Chinese labor was even more justified in the white community's mind after plague infected San Francisco.

White San Franciscans, like the Victorian British, prided themselves on an "ethic of progress."[19] San Francisco was a major shipping port in the Pacific, its mining magnates had poured money into building an aesthetically pleasing urban façade, and the city had a thriving financial district. Mayor Phelan wanted the rest of America and the world to view San Francisco as the "Paris of the Pacific." The ruling white population took the credit for San Francisco's economic and cultural success. Later when Mayor Phelan ran for the U. S. Senate under the slogan, "Keep California White," he reinforced this view of white superiority.[20]

When white San Franciscans heard about the Hawaiian plague in 1899, the reaction was denial that it could ever reach their climate-proof and sophisticated city.[21] White San Franciscans' sense of success, like the British in Hong Kong, rendered the belief that plague ever could enter their beautiful port impossible. Like the Chinese plague victims in Hong Kong, those in San Francisco were the target of ruling whites' projected disdain. The concentration of the disease initially in Chinatown provided easy fodder for scapegoating. And Chinese immorality was once again offered as the cause of plague. Two months after the first case of plague there, the *San Francisco Morning Call* gave its opinion about the origin of the disease in its town. The editorial blamed the very existence of Chinatown: "so long as it stands so long will there be a menace of the appearance in San Francisco of every form of disease, plague, and pestilence which Asiatic filth and vice generate."[22]

Chinese scapegoating in San Francisco was not a new phenomenon. In an 1885 City Hall report that analyzed Chinatown's public health, the Chinese were believed to carry "the virus of immorality" that was ultimately responsible for infectious diseases such as tuberculosis and leprosy.[23] So when plague arrived in San Francisco in 1900, the white community's disdain of the disease's threats to its own sense of progress was conveniently projected onto the less prominent ethnic group that already posed a financial threat.

Chinese immorality, of course, did not cause plague. By 1900 the world knew that the bacterial cause of plague had been discovered. However, the first scientist in charge of addressing and controlling plague in San Francisco, Joseph Kinyoun, faced skepticism from the medical community there even though he isolated the newly discovered bacterium from dead plague victims in Chinatown. In 1900 San Francisco, "the new bacteriology was still [viewed as] a form of black magic."[24] And so it was easy to blame Chinese culture for the appearance of the disease.

But not for long. In early 1905, San Francisco was perplexed when three Italians in the same family contracted the pneumonic form of plague and died. They had no contact with Chinatown, where the other 120 cases emerged. These deaths undermined any theory that Chinese immorality alone caused plague. A further blow to this Chinese immorality theory came in the form of a destructive 8.3 Richter scale earthquake in April 1906. The rats unsettled by this earthquake were quite active in districts outside of Chinatown. Rupert Blue, who was in charge of controlling the disease near the end of the first epidemic in San Francisco, ordered the construction of cement basements in Chinatown during 1903–04. After the 1906 earthquake, the rats could not infiltrate these residents' homes. As 1907 closed, there were 136 people infected with the disease and 73 had died; the majority of them were *not* Chinese.[25]

Rat extermination ultimately abetted the departure of acute *Yersinia pestis* infection from San Francisco. Blue spearheaded a huge rat extermination program after the earthquake, and by November 1907 his rat-catching team collected 13,000 rats per week.[26] By October 1908, there had been no more human cases of the disease for eight months. The Chinese could no longer serve as the scapegoat because this outbreak barely touched them. Scientific interventions, not racist ones, squelched the disease in the city. Blue explained to a reporter that "plague is no respecter of individuals or places."[27] Indeed, the disease caused by *Yersinia pestis*, at least in its bubonic form, is transmitted by the fleas on infected rats and not by cultural differences.

The incidence of *Yersinia pestis* infection in the twentieth century remained low overall. After the San Francisco epidemics, the next notable one occurred in Los Angeles in 1924. Forty people contracted the pneumonic form of the disease and approximately 30 people died.[28] The disease then became endemic in the southwestern United States, where an average of 12 cases per year still occurs today. Other countries, including Brazil, Congo, Madagascar (where a resistant strain erupted in 1995), Peru, and Vietnam, also currently experience minor outbreaks.[29]

By far the worst outbreak of *Yersinia pestis* in the twentieth century was in India in 1994, although this one pales in comparison with the epidemics of past centuries. The statistics on the number of cases and deaths in India varied daily from news source to news source, but *The New York Times* provided thorough daily coverage. The first cases of the disease were on September 24, 1994, in Surat.[30] Within the week, Indian officials suspected a case rise of 1,000–2,000.[31] The country was declared free of the disease one month later, with the final death toll at less than 60 people. The World Health Organization surmised that no more than 300 people in India contracted the bacterium that caused both the bubonic and pneumonic forms of the disease in a total population of 920 million.[32]

Yet in spite of these sobering statistics and in spite of an age when antibiotics certainly existed—tetracycline quickly reached even the most remote Indian villages after the first cases were reported—this outbreak provoked extreme and classic reactions to plague. The label of plague persisted in spite of the fact that the bacterial cause of the disease had been known for a century. On the first day of the reported cases, *The New York Times* headlined the disease's debut as "Deadly Plague Outbreak." However, the death toll was only 24 people in a population of hundreds of millions.[33]

People panicked. Approximately 200,000 residents left Surat after the disease's pneumonic appearance was announced. The Health Ministry in India, however, responded rationally by sending millions of tablets of tetracycline to the residents of Surat so they could take them at the first sign of infection. This Ministry also administered DDT, a powerful pesticide, in order to kill the fleas that potentially carry the bacterium. One health official even said, "there is no cause for alarm."[34] Indeed only 24 people had died and these officials were attempting to prevent a massive epidemic. But deep in the psyche of the Indian people were memories of the late-nineteenth-century Bombay outbreak that did not leave the country for more than 20 years and killed more than 10 million people. Reporters apparently appealed to these memories.

By the end of the first week in September, the number of deaths rose from 24 to 47, with hundreds more being treated. The death toll was actually quite small. But in a September 29 article, the disease was described in the headline as "Return of the Plague."[35] It is not just *a* plague but *the* plague of yore. This descriptor for a minor outbreak of the disease unites it with other major plague outbreaks over the centuries. Furthermore, this article opens with a description of the disease's "magical" reappearance here in India: "Like a nightmare returning from the Middle Ages, an epidemic of plague has struck India."[36] In reality, the disease did not appear in India until the early twentieth century, and it only emerged now in 1994 because an earthquake shook nearby Latur, which produced flooding that unsettled the rat population. The author of this article also reminds the reader of the many devastating plague outbreaks in past centuries, including the earlier twentieth-century one in India. By creating this context, the author solidifies the position of this later Indian outbreak in the narrative genealogy of plague.

The articles stopped coming after one month of this minor outbreak in India, but plague has survived in other literature and film throughout the twentieth century. Herman Hesse's 1930 novel *Narcissus and Goldmund* devotes time to plague in his turn of the nineteenth to twentieth-century setting. He provides plague platitudes, or stock images of and reactions to the disease, from earlier centuries, such as death carts with heaps of corpses upon them, the digging of plague pits, and unburied corpses after the pits were filled. Reactions of fear prevail when Goldmund and Robert are denied entrance to several towns because outsiders were thought to carry the plague. The culture of death appears in a dance macabre painting in a cloister's fresco that depicts people from different ranks of society who are taunted by skeletons playing instruments.[37]

Albert Camus' 1948 novel, *The Plague*, falls into a medieval tradition, on the one hand, by adopting the historical "chronicle" as its narrative frame. The narrator, Dr. Bernard Rieux, announces that he is a historian writing about plague in 1940s Oran.[38] Camus employs the plague label for the disease caused by *Yersinia pestis*, but treats it as a medical illness and not a moral one throughout the novel. Rieux sends for plague serum, not priests, that arrives the day after the quarantine for people living in the same house with the sick goes into effect. Eventually, the entire town will be under a quarantine order in order to halt the disease's spread beyond its borders.

Camus certainly captures more classic responses to plague, most notably in the character of the Jesuit priest, Father Paneloux. His sermon to the Oran townspeople, after the first month of plague with the death toll nearing 500 people per week, is something right out of the Middle Ages. He preaches that human sin in general is responsible for this divine punishment and reverts to more medieval nomenclature for the disease; it is "the scourge of God" and "pestilence."[39] He also forges this quite severe outbreak in Oran into plague history by reminding the congregation of the plague that struck the Pharaoh in Egypt and by discussing a medieval French chronicler of the disease who said the disease was an indication of eternal damnation.

Other traditional responses to the disease, such as flight after the town quarantine is imposed and hedonism that takes the form of excessive late night drunkenness and public fighting, appear from time to time in Camus' work. Plague-induced despair, however, reaches new heights. The townspeople usually enjoy the heat of the summer, but during this plague-ridden season the "plague had killed all colors, vetoed pleasure."[40] Camus adds to the centuries-long plague narrative by fusing modern existential angst with the traditional reaction of despair. As day after day passes with the parades of corpses through the streets, the people might have "retained the attitudes of sadness and suffering, but they had ceased to feel their sting."[41] A feeling of no pleasure is despair, but a new level of despair is reached when one cannot even feel that no pleasure is felt.

After the publication of Camus' novel, some Hollywood movies that focused on plague, in particular Elia Kazan's *Panic in the Streets* and Ingmar Bergman's *The Seventh Seal*, were produced in the 1950s.[42] Although Kazan's title and opening staccato music create the impression of "panic," this movie that has plague as its main subject approaches the disease with rationality. It unfolds as both a murder and disease mystery when a murder victim in twentieth-century New Orleans is discovered to have been infected with *Yersinia pestis*. Dr. Reed, played by Richard Widmark, of the U.S. Health Services Department becomes instrumental in working with the police captain to swiftly and methodically find the murderer(s), who were exposed to the infection, within the next 48 hours in order to thwart the spread of the disease.

Although Kazan's characters in the movie consistently refer to the disease as *plague*, typical responses to the disease are not prevalent. Admittedly, there is some disdain of the disease's presence in the ship captain's persistent denial of the plague/murder victim on his ship when Dr. Reed and the police captain investigate the vessel that brought the man to America. And there is flight when one of the mayor's officials quickly decides to take his children to their grandmother's home outside of the city before the murderer, Blackey, is caught by officials. But there is no reference to a divine source of plague in this movie, and no wholehearted attempt to create a human one. Immorality and plague are not Kazan's subjects. Instead, Kazan presents a rational response to the disease: a swift official effort to contain the disease and conceal the few cases so that there is *not* a "panic in the streets."

Seven years later with the release of Ingmar Bergman's *The Seventh Seal* we are transported back to the Middle Ages and to quite classic responses to plague. A knight and his squire have just returned from many years of crusading in the Holy Land only to find their country "ravaged by the Black Plague."[43] Bergman's setting has historical accuracy. In 1349, bubonic plague was in Norway.[44] At other points in the movie, the disease is simply called "plague" and most notably the "Black Death." Bergman's work understandably, yet anachronistically, uses this popular term for the disease that was coined in sixteenth-century Sweden.[45]

Back in Bergman's Middle Ages, death is ubiquitous. The knight and squire come upon a decaying corpse that sits upright on a rock as they journey home; they also pass through deserted villages. The figure of Death is a pervasive presence that the knight plays chess with in order to win his own life. The horror of death is captured by the painter in the church where the knight and the squire stop. "The Dance of Death" is the subject of this painting because, according to the artist, "this is what life is now."[46] The painter also reveals the popular medieval belief in divine causes of plague when he explains that people in this country inflict bodily self-punishment in order to atone for God's anger. Flagellants, a radical Christian group that spread throughout Europe in the Middle Ages, believed that lashing themselves with whips would appease God and stop the plague. They also did not hesitate to blame the Jews for plague, especially in Germany.

Bergman also frames his movie with an apocalyptic theme. In the beginning of the film, the narrator discusses the opening of the seventh seal before we even meet the knight and the squire. At one point, villagers eating dinner comment on the swiftness of death from plague and say "it is judgment day."[47] The primary survivors of the opening of the seventh seal in this movie are the happily married actors who at one point extended their hospitality to the knight. They are aptly named Mary and Joseph and have a newborn son who does not need to be named.

Diseases caused by organisms other than the bacterium *Yersinia pestis* were labeled plagues in the twentieth century, namely the influenza virus. The 1918 influenza outbreak acquired the name "Spanish flu" after it swept Spain and infected the king there in February 1918. According to Gina Kolata, "it swept the globe in months," and visited America in September of this year, killing a half a million people. Worldwide the disease killed anywhere from 20 to more than 100 million people.[48] Actually, "the flu killed more people in 24 weeks than AIDS has killed in 24 years."[49] Not surprisingly, Kolata has no qualms about calling the influenza epidemic a "plague" throughout her book.[50]

Influenza also has been depicted fictionally as plague. The title of Katherine Anne Porter's 1939 short story, "Pale Horse, Pale Rider," alludes to John's Book of the Apocalypse.[51] When the fourth seal is broken, Death rides out on a horse, murdering people with his weapon of plague. While working as a reporter in Denver, Porter contracted influenza in 1918 and recovered, unlike her fiancé. In the story, Miranda and Adam walk down a street and discuss the new disease that is making so many people sick. Miranda describes it as "plague, something out of the Middle Ages." And when she catches it, her landlady wants her removed from the building because "this is a plague, a plague, my God."[52]

Like Porter's short story earlier in the twentieth century, Stephen King's 1978 novel, *The Stand*, focuses on a deadly flu epidemic, although his fictional account is not based on a factual event.[53] King's novel, however, reiterates familiar plague motifs on the verge of AIDS' appearance in the United States. King forges a relationship between the "super flu" outbreak of 1980 America and plague.[54] This flu strikes quickly and kills people everywhere, creating a virtual land of corpses. *Plague* becomes an umbrella term in this novel for any infectious disease, including this "super flu." The Centers for Disease Control (CDC) is known as the "Plague Center in Atlanta."[55]

King also explores apocalyptic motifs in his novel that form a relationship between flu and plague even more. Frequently, characters view this virulent new strain of influenza as a harbinger of the end of the world. Some type of Judgment Day seems imminent in the novel when the prophet Mother Abigail leads the "good" people, who are immune to the plague, to Boulder, Colorado, in order to "stand" against the "evil" ones who follow the devil Randall Flagg.

Porter's and King's plagues are highly infectious diseases with a high mortality rate but they have a viral cause and not a divine one. Also, Porter and King do not offer any scapegoats for their plagues. If AIDS had to enter the scene as a plague in 1981 America, Porter and King laid the groundwork for the disease joining this non-*Yersinia pestis* thread of the global plague narrative where there are no divine or human causes. Instead, AIDS enters like a medieval miasma that does not dissipate even after scientists identify its viral cause a few years later.

PART III

The Emergence of AIDS

CHAPTER 6

The Making of a Plague (1981–1986)

And then there was Larry. When I began working in oncology in Manhattan in 1986, AIDS patients always appeared on my unit because of their accompanying cancer diagnoses and because no one knew where else they belonged. What I did not expect was to encounter patients with AIDS on the VIP unit I moonlighted on occasionally after my regular shift was over.

The supervisor of the VIP unit was a fellow Pennsylvanian whom I met one weekend when she covered my unit. She enticed me to work overtime on her floor because it would be an "easy shift" in comparison to the intense care we delivered to quite ill cancer patients. And the shifts *were* easy—in fact, too easy. I was not dealing with complicated chemotherapy regimens, nausea, high temperatures, and exhausted families. Instead, I was at hand to apply fresh ice packs to patients with facial lifts and most importantly serve crushed ice—not cubed, as one of my patients reminded me—with the evening orange juice rounds.

One evening during the spring of 1987, I was assigned to a patient there with a planned admission for later in my shift. The KS diagnosis was surprising here. Even more intriguing was his esteemed status as one of the first people in the United States diagnosed with this cancer in the late 1970s before anyone knew the ultimate viral culprit.

Before Larry arrived there were beautiful lilies delivered to his room. The auxiliary staff arranged them just so for our next VIP's stay. Around 7:00 a man donned in black stepped off the elevator and approached the nurse's station. I assumed he was a visitor with a question until I spotted one faintly purplish lesion on his left ear. "Good evening. I am Larry B., and I am scheduled for room 891." I introduced myself and informed him of the lovely flower arrangement already delivered to his room. "I sent them to myself," he said.

Larry was educated, sophisticated, and not wanting economically. He boasted about the length of time he had KS and about his famous oncologist who had managed to nudge it into remission three or four times before. He was also filled with a little pride over the fact that he had this cancer before terms like "retrovirus" became a part of our medical lexicon. I asked him how he felt when all of the AIDS talk began. "Well, a little scared but mostly intrigued." That was Larry: a lot of intellectualizing with a splatter of emotion. It would be difficult later in the year even to get him to admit how much pain he had when the KS infiltrated his mouth, lungs, and intestines.

I wondered why he was not admitted to my oncology unit. "I prefer it here," he explained: "the environment and food are so much better." After all, this was the VIP floor that catered to the more esoteric needs of its denizens. I knew the direction in which his disease was headed and I wanted him to know that the care on the oncology ward was provided by nurses with expert knowledge and experience who could address his needs. Interferon was ordered for his KS and it usually caused high fevers, night sweats, and general malaise.

Larry also admitted that he liked the fact that his diagnosis was more "hidden" on the VIP unit. Of course, he meant his cancer diagnosis. He had not come to terms with the progression of his cancer and an admission to my unit would have held that mirror up to his face. On the VIP floor, he was just one diagnosis among the face-lifts, skin cancer removals, and nervous breakdowns. I suspected that he was equally concerned with keeping the AIDS diagnosis "hidden." His medical chart on this unit actually only presented his cancer as the diagnosis. I had to dig pretty deep in a doctor's note to find his HIV antibody status.

Prior to the development of the HIV antibody test in 1985, Larry just had cancer but now his cancer was an AIDS-defining diagnosis. We talked about how this new relationship with HIV made his cancer more public. In recent years, he seemed to relish in his ability to shock people during times when his KS had recurred and become more visible. Especially in elevators, he would purposively position himself in the middle of a staring crowd and announce: "Yes. I have AIDS. You better exit quickly." I began to understand that beneath his poised façade of intellectualism, there was a person who had experienced a fair amount of discrimination. His reaction to this was his elevator performances and his firm commitment to be admitted only to the VIP unit where his cancer and HIV status were simply glossed over in favor of four-star hotel services.

The next day I worked on my unit and talked to my supervisor about how Larry belonged with us. Of course, she agreed. After work, I went to visit Larry in his ritzy room and I met his parents. They were really only willing to discuss the cancer diagnosis. I used their interest in that diagnosis as leverage for my presentation regarding the high quality of care we oncology nurses could provide for him in the future—only if he needed it, of course.

A few months later, near the end of the summer, when the sweltering heat and humidity drives most New Yorkers elsewhere, the charge nurse on my unit showed me the name of the patient being admitted and asked if it was the same Larry I cared for on the VIP unit. I smiled but only for a brief moment. I realized that I was successful in convincing him to come to my unit, but I knew he was probably far more ill than he was when I saw him last.

This time, he arrived via wheelchair and had lost about 20 pounds from his already too-slim frame. The interferon was not working and he would need more aggressive chemotherapy for the KS lesions that now erupted daily on his face. After a month—yes, he stayed longer than that and was not discharged in a wheelchair—the cancer would invade even his gums, peeking out through his teeth on the left upper side of his mouth. Now, I began to work overtime on my unit. Shift after double shift, I grew to know this man, his partner, his family, and his few remaining friends. It was always hard for his mother to accept that her good looking, successful, and smart son "turned into a homosexual" (that is how she explained it) during his stay away at college in the early 1970s. It was even harder for his father, who never said too much in his room. But both of them were there every day at his bedside.

Larry and I became friends, not something I am supposed to admit or let happen as a nurse. Friendships with patients make it difficult to maintain healthy barriers and advocate more objectively for them. It can result in what I have experienced for more than 20 years since Larry's death in the fall of 1987: painful joy every time I smell a lily. Yes, the lilies were always in this room, too. I especially enjoyed our 11 P.M. conversations when my other patients were settled for the night. He opened up more about what it meant to have AIDS. He revealed that in the past few months before this hospitalization, he faced rejection from friends who stopped inviting him to dinner and simply stopped calling, and from clients who stopped buying the clothes he designed. He grew to realize that some nurses, doctors, and even x-ray technicians did not want to care for him *because* of his diagnosis. A guarded form of discrimination manifested itself in some of the medical staff who did not touch him during bath time—figure that one out—did not listen to his lungs with a stethoscope even though the KS found a new home there, and banged the x-ray machine against his bedside rails, not once but several times, when no one was there to witness this hostile act.

On his deathbed, Larry became fully aware of the discrimination he had been experiencing because of his diagnosis, and I was growing with him in this awareness. One month before Larry died, I read a review of a book by San Francisco journalist Randy Shilts, who chronicled the AIDS epidemic to date. I was a little surprised when I went to my local bookstore (a chain) only to discover that they did not carry *And the Band Played On*. As I was getting ready to ask the clerk when they would have the book, a man next to me said, "Don't hold your breath, honey. I've looked in all of the major bookstores, too. Only the gay bookshop on Christopher Street downtown carries it." Perhaps this was another form of guarded discrimination. There was no ban on Randy Shilts' book; in fact, it was reviewed favorably, but major bookstores were simply not carrying it *yet*.

I had never been on Christopher Street before. I had only moved to the city a little more than a year earlier and there was still so much to discover. I had read about the Stonewall riots that happened on this street, but I did not fully understand the significance of this event or the liberation movement spurred by it. I entered the bookshop and the owner asked me if I was looking for something in particular. He pointed me to the shelf where Shilts' book was propped, and I explained to him that the mainstream bookstores were not carrying it. He smiled, "I know, but we have plenty of copies here." He asked me if I minded telling him *why* I was so interested in the book. "I take care of AIDS patients and I want to learn more." "Thank you," he said, before I exited his shop.

And the Band Played On explained to me what I had witnessed with my previous AIDS patients and what I was witnessing now as I cared for Larry: discrimination against people who had a terrible disease. Shilts' book made, for the first time in the infancy of my career, taking care of AIDS patients a political act and a duty. I shared this book with Larry and his partner as I read it. And then as I wrapped Larry's body in the early morning hour after I came on duty—I still like to believe that the night shift nurse really was too busy to perform postmortem care—I knew that I had no other choice but to transfer to the newly created unit for AIDS patients. I did one month later.

In the five years before I cared for Larry, AIDS inherited some fairly ugly connotations. A close review of *how* AIDS was described by scientists, journalists, and artists from 1981 to 1986 will assist in understanding the making of a plague that resulted in the discrimination Larry and others experienced. One would think that the first official report of this immunological disorder in the CDC's *Morbidity and Mortality Weekly Report* would be free of any bias toward anyone with the disease. After all, this is the CDC's official scientific tally and summary of new and existing diseases, including infectious ones. But scientific writings, like we witnessed with historical ones in earlier centuries, cannot achieve complete objectivity. Objectivity is relative to the cultural position of the author and the reader.

The *MMWR's* first report of what would later become an AIDS-related pneumonia was on June 5, 1981.[1] *Pneumocystis carinii* pneumonia, as it was known then, would be renamed *Pneumocystis jirveci* in 2002 when the microorganism was thought to be more fungal than protozoan in its features, but today it retains the acronym PCP. The CDC's initial presentation of PCP made it seem like it was a specifically gay male disease. Before each of the five cases in this report was discussed, the young men were described as "all active homosexuals," two of whom had "frequent homosexual contacts with various partners."[2] It indeed was curious in 1981 that anyone would have PCP without chemotherapy or organ transplant therapy that induced immuno-suppression. But why did the CDC characterize these five cases based on their sexual orientation? Would "heterosexual" have accompanied these case presentations if that had been the sexual orientation of these men?

It is understandable that the CDC was attempting to make connections between the type and frequency of sexual activity and the occurrence of PCP—actually a quite prescient epidemiological theory in 1981. But when the Editorial Note following this report attempted to justify the significance of the cases' sexual orientation by suggesting that there is "an association between some aspect of a homosexual lifestyle or disease acquired through sexual contact and *Pneumocystis* pneumonia in this population," the gay nature of this pneumonia is reinforced.[3] At first I thought there was a typo-graphical error in this sentence with the conjunction "or," and it was meant to read that there was an association between a homosexual lifestyle "and" a disease acquired through any type of sexual contact that could expose one to PCP. My own cultural position as a reader explains my interpretation. Reading the sentence as it was printed with "or" makes it seem like there is a specifically "homosexual disease" that exposes one to PCP, as opposed to reading "and" in the sentence, which would make the "sexual contact disease" free from sexual orientation.

Why exactly would a *homosexual* as opposed to a *heterosexual* disease acquired through sexual contact make one more vulnerable to PCP? Further-more, what disease infects *only* homosexuals? An epidemiological dichotomy was suggested here between homosexual and heterosexual diseases, and thus PCP began its trajectory as a gay male disease. And the label did stick. I cared for a patient in 1986 with mesothelioma—a type of lung cancer from asbestos exposure—who contracted PCP after an intense course of immunosuppres-sive chemotherapy. He was embarrassed to tell his wife that he had, as he phrased it, "that gay pneumonia."

The second *MMWR* report released one month later discussed what would become an AIDS-defining cancer, Kaposi's sarcoma.[4] This report also forged a direct relationship between sexual orientation and this new disease.

"Twenty-six *homosexual* men" were diagnosed with KS within the last 30 months and, like PCP, this appearance had not been seen previously in gay men.[5] KS usually affects elderly men of Mediterranean descent, young adults in certain parts of Africa, and transplant patients. The appearance of KS in homosexual men was "considered highly unusual" by the CDC at this time, but it was also unusual that the sexual orientation of these elderly men and Africans had never been considered, as this report admits.[6] Nonetheless, this scientific discourse that aligned sexual orientation or, as the CDC put it, "sexual preference,"[7] with cancer paved the way for the possibility of blame to be assigned to those with KS. If one could get the cancer because one "prefers" to be gay, then one could prevent the cancer by choosing not to be gay.

The New York Times reported the appearance of KS on the same day that the CDC released its report. This newspaper is known for its high-caliber reporting and was invaluable for its coverage of AIDS in a city that bore the brunt of the disease's casualties; however, objectivity in journalistic writing is relative to the cultural position of the writer and of the reader, as well. This article's author is Lawrence K. Altman, not only a journalist but a medical doctor, so we have the advantage of an expert in both fields covering the epidemic. But the cancer was also presented as a "gay" one, the article's title being "Rare Cancer Seen in 41 Homosexuals."[8] Altman's statistics for the number of homosexuals affected by KS differ from the CDC's 26 cases because he based his numbers on an interview with a local physician. He acknowledged, however, that the CDC was supposed to release its official report on the day of his own article's publication with the 26 cases of KS. Why didn't the newspaper wait for the definitive CDC report before publishing Altman's article? Altman's report of even more cases had the effect of inciting more anxiety and concern over this cancer's appearance in a population untouched by it before, as did his comment that KS had a "sudden appearance" in these men.[9] The CDC described a more gradual appearance of KS over 30 months with fewer cases.

Altman's article also details the sexual practices of these men with KS. According to a local doctor he interviewed, most of these men with KS engaged in "multiple and frequent sexual encounters with different partners."[10] But these are not enough details. Some of them had "10 sexual encounters each night up to four times a week."[11] In addition, these gay men used drugs "to heighten sexual pleasure" and carried many infectious diseases, including hepatitis B and CMV.[12] In this seemingly "objective" journalistic account of the first KS cases, gay men appear to be wild, sex-crazed infectious vectors who, not surprisingly, have a cancer usually seen in a different demographic. This depiction of KS tapped into prejudicial sentiments against gay men in a country that was deeply engaged in an ongoing clash between more secular mores unleashed during the late 1960s and more conservative ones reacting against them.

The civil rights movement throughout the 1960s was comprised of different social groups that fought for recognition and ultimately acceptance by our society at large. African Americans, American Indians, women, and gays, to name a few groups, were propelled into political action against established American institutions that did not recognize their rights as diverse groups, and in most instances treated them with guarded or open discrimination.

Gay men took political action at this time in order to be recognized as a distinct sexual group, like heterosexuals. Medical science after all had viewed homosexuality as a psychological disorder, and the gay community was no longer willing to accept this view. The medical establishment viewed homosexuality as a "pathological disorder" that could be "cured" with psychoanalysis. On the other hand, the homophile movement refused to accept this view by arguing "that sexual orientation was inborn" and therefore incapable of being cured.[13] Larry Kramer's main character, Ned Weeks, in *The Destiny of Me* is a testament to the years of psychotherapy gay men had to endure when the goal was to cure sexual orientation. The effects on this character's psyche, such as a certain degree of self-hatred, were damaging for many gay people who were also subjected to the hope of a cure during this time period.[14]

Throughout the 1960s, the gay liberation movement began to flourish in response to discriminatory views and actions against them. In 1964, the San Francisco police's persistent raids of gay bars provoked the creation of the Society for Individual Rights, which according to Martin Duberman, became "the largest homophile organization in the country."[15] In the late 1960s, the Stonewall Inn on Christopher Street in New York City's Greenwich Village had opened its doors to gay men who could comfortably dance there. Although the bar was raided by police less than other gay bars in the city, when a raid occurred without the usual warning to the owners on June 27, 1968, the patrons fought back for the first time. Outside, drag queens jumped out of the police wagon; some fought back physically, and others sang and danced in a chorus line proudly announcing their identities as queens.[16] Protests ensued in front of the bar the next night and people wrote, "Legalize gay bars" and "Support gay power" on the boarded windows.[17] These slogans captured the significance of the Stonewall riots: a formal rejection of discrimination against gay people and a public demand for equality.

It was this importance that I did not understand the first time I went to Christopher Street to buy Shilts' book, which incidentally was sold to me by the owner and founder of the Oscar Wilde Memorial Bookshop, Craig Rodwell. He was there during the Stonewall riots and helped organize the first Gay Pride March in 1970 that commemorated the anniversary of the riots. This parade remains a staple of New York City life every June. The riots also inspired the formation of more activist groups, such as the Gay Liberation Front, that included lesbians who often felt underrepresented in other gay political groups.

One of the most significant influences of the gay rights movement in general was the removal of homosexuality as a mental disorder from *The Diagnostic and Statistical Manual of Mental Disorders* (*DSM*) in 1973. This manual, now in its fourth edition, catalogues psychological disorders and details their accompanying symptoms. Homosexuality was no longer classified as a mental disorder in 1973, but unfortunately it was reclassified by the *DSM* as a "sexual orientation disturbance." Finally in the 1986 edition, it was removed as a "disturbance."[18] But at least by the early 1970s gay people were no longer considered mentally ill by the medical establishment, a view that certainly facilitated some consideration of gay rights.

The civil rights atmosphere of the late 1960s also inspired people to find their religious identities. Many people sought a renewed, personal relationship with a divine being or other-worldly realm. An evangelical Protestant movement emerged in counterpoint to the New Age movement. Evangelicals, in particular, valued "the individual's experience of grace, and the personal discovery of one's own salvation."[19] Their stress on a more "personal" relationship with God over the group's relationship morphed into an influential religion a decade later that was "far more likely to divide than to integrate."[20] By 1986, 32 percent of all Americans considered themselves "born again or evangelical Christians."[21]

In tandem with this religious group's ascendancy to popularity was a more conservative political ideology in the United States. President Nixon's "conservative revolution," during his reelection campaign in 1972, exerted some influence a decade later.[22] Nixon promulgated less federal government involvement and a shift in power to the states and even the private sector. By the time Ronald Reagan campaigned for his presidency in 1980, the New Right became a fait accompli. Reagan worked closely with evangelical Christian organizations, such as the Moral Majority,[23] and his policies on AIDS research and funding throughout the 1980s became a testament to his more conservative political and religious beliefs.

It would seem that a religious and political ideology that denounces big government and seeks to uphold individual rights, such as religious practices, gun ownership, and the accumulation of personal wealth unfettered by federal taxes, would value individual rights in general, including a woman's right to decide whether or not to carry a fetus to term, and for anyone's right to be in a gay or straight relationship with or without marriage. Instead, the "nuclear family" not only became the symbol of the New Right's platform but produced programs that, as Cindy Patton points out, "aimed to reverse the trends that were perceived to have attacked" this family.[24] The supposed "attackers" would include women who divorce and abort, and, of course, the gay community.

The New Right's paradoxical espousal of some individual freedoms and the denial of others might be understood as projected disdain. Like some Catholics in the Middle Ages who were disgusted with and threatened by their own Church's weaknesses and consequently projected this disdain onto the Jews, the religious thread of the New Right in the early 1980s might have been disgusted by their own needs for personal salvation and projected this self-disdain onto groups like the gay community, who did not seek this type of rescue. Gay relationships certainly did not fit the New Right's mold of the nuclear family, an image that they clung to in order to abet personal salvation and grace.

AIDS emerged in this cultural climate in which more secular and politically liberal social groups existed at one pole of American life and more religious and politically conservative social groups existed at the other. For very different reasons, the ideology of both poles influenced the construction of AIDS as a plague in the early 1980s. This construction built upon the initial descriptions of the disease in mid-1981 as specifically "homosexual," and it continued to be described as a gay disease even though non-gay people contracted it. A prominent medical journal article titled "Pneumocystis carinni Pneumonia and Mucosal Candidiasis in Previously Healthy Homosexual Men," near the end of 1981 presented the disease as a gay male one. The lead author, Michael Gottlieb, M.D., who identified the first cases of PCP for the CDC, here focused on four more men with this pneumonia.[25] Again, explicit details of the sexual activities of these sick men are provided, and their behavior is described as a salient feature in contracting it. There is no overt judgment by the authors about the sexual habits of these men; rather the goal is to isolate a common variable that results in the disease. The authors conclude that "a sexually transmitted infectious agent" is the cause of the disease, which certainly proves to be the case a few years later.[26] However, this proposed agent apparently is *not* restricted to the male homosexual community but the article's title would have us believe otherwise. In an addendum note submitted after the article was under consideration for publication, the authors admit that this syndrome also was documented "in two exclusively heterosexual men."[27] And a few months before this article's publication, a newspaper article reported a woman with PCP in the 53 cases collected so far.[28] Perhaps the authors of this *New England Journal of Medicine* article should have amended their title in order to more accurately reflect all of the groups with this disease.

The following year, reporting on the syndrome persists in describing AIDS as specifically gay in nature. A newspaper article in May 1982 calls it a "new homosexual disorder," and on several occasions refers to it by its short-lived acronym, GRID (Gay Related Immune Deficiency). Yet the author of this article recognizes that "researchers call it AID for acquired immunodeficiency disease," which has been found in "heterosexual women"—13 to be exact— "and bisexual and heterosexual men."[29] This is far from being an exclusively "new homosexual disorder." Again, the journalist here highlights the sexual promiscuity of the gay men with the disease, which has the effect of inciting prejudicial feelings about gays in people who harbor them baseline. This journalist, however, does not judge gay sexual practices nor present them as morally reprehensible. This article, like Dr. Gottlieb's, presents AIDS as an almost exclusively homosexual disease in an effort to investigate its cause in one highly affected sexual group as opposed to exploring sexual acts among different groups.

These presumably scientific presentations of AIDS give us a gay disease that also begins to be surrounded by plague discourse. For example, the disease was often presented as an affliction. In the summer of 1981 when the first cases of PCP and KS were reported, one article reported that "two rare diseases have *struck* more than 100 homosexual men in the United States in recent months."[30] By May 1982, the disorder was "*afflicting* at least 335 people" who are "primarily male homosexuals."[31] Like Apollo with his arrows aimed at the Greek army in Homer's ancient poem, this immunological disorder targets gay men.

This affliction becomes stealthier in other reports by 1983. The number of Americans with PCP and KS had grown from the original handfuls to more than 1,000 with almost half of them dead.[32] One extensive article written in February 1983 covered the disease's impact on non-gay groups but highlights its gay nature. A picture of a Gay Men's Health Crisis conference—an organization founded in the early 1980s by a few gay men, including Larry Kramer, in New York City for the sole purpose of supporting people with AIDS—captures the participants' grave concern with the disease. Their serious and saddened countenances are deepened by the caption that describes the disease as a perpetrator that has brought them together. AIDS "*stalks* the homosexual community."[33] Later in this article, AIDS turns into a bogeyman who specifically taunts gay men. The journalist ominously declares that "the specter of AIDS haunts every member of the homosexual community."[34] This is similar to the view of the fourteenth-century Welsh poet Gethin, who saw the bubonic plague as a phantom that haunts his entire community.

AIDS was not only described as a "gay affliction" but as a "gay plague" in several different sources. In an August 1982 *Newsweek* update, the disease is called the less sexually charged "Acquired Immunodeficiency Syndrome" in the article's text, but the title describes it as a "homosexual plague" that "strikes new victims."[35] The lid obviously could not be sealed tightly enough on the gay community's exclusive ability to carry this disease when the authors proclaim that "the homosexual plague has started spilling over into the general population."[36] As early as 1982, AIDS began to gain plague status because it was supposedly spreading into non-gay populations. When plague is a disease, it is highly infectious—as this article would have us believe about AIDS—but only 505 cases had been reported in the United States with a total population of more than 230 million.[37] AIDS actually was not highly infectious at this time. A virologist declared in early 1983, "We are not dealing with the Black Plague. You're not going to get AIDS from toilet seats or eating in restaurants."[38]

Yet the 40 percent mortality rate of AIDS at this time certainly facilitated a view of it as a plague because it killed so many of those who contracted it. But why was it a *gay* one? In effect, labeling it as such places responsibility in the gay population for the disease's spread. In 1982 the disease was presented as a plague with a gay origin that is now spreading *from* infected gays *to* uninfected non-gays (the "general population").[39] Cultural constructions of diseases as plague, especially *Yersinia pestis* disease, usually are accompanied by discrimination against certain marginalized groups of people like the Jews and the Chinese. The labeling of AIDS as a *gay plague* was only the beginning of fomenting blame and hatred for gay men with AIDS that in time would transfer to others with the disease.

These references to AIDS as gay plague in the mainstream media fueled more conservative believers to have no qualms about calling the disease a plague even after HIV was determined to be its viral cause by 1984. The plague label in the hands of the New Right stems from a place of judgment, and even downright hatred, of homosexuals. The title of Lawrence Lockman's 1986 book, *The AIDS Epidemic: a Citizen's Guide to Protecting Your Family and Community from the Gay Plague,* alone forecasts its moral tenor. This treatise is an argument against any acceptance of the gay community, and it is an endorsement of their culpability for the existence and spread of AIDS. In splashes of red, a warning from the publisher appears on the first page lambasting the sexual activities of homosexuals as "extremely filthy and disgusting as well as unhealthy."[40] The reader needs to be warned because Lockman feels compelled later on to give explicit details of their sexual practices. These sordid details are supposed to serve as his proof of the unhealthy nature of homosexuality. This vilification leads to Lockman calling the disease "the gay plague."[41] Gay sex violates Lockman's conservative belief system and can only result in AIDS (plague).

Lockman extends the gay plague label to even heterosexuals whom he believes contracted the disease through non-traditional and non-conservative sexual practices. "Gay denotes swinging heterosexuals too," he announces, because police officers used the term "gay" to denote promiscuous prostitutes. These heterosexuals, therefore, become "carriers of the gay plague of AIDS" because they do not fit the New Right's ideas about acceptable sexual practices within the confines of the nuclear family.[42]

Members of the gay community viewed AIDS as a gay plague also, but not because they objected to being gay. In the early 1980s this community was devastated by the sheer number of its members contracting and dying from the disease. Larry Kramer's powerful article from March 1983, "1,112 and Counting," tallies the number of AIDS cases thus far, the majority of whom were gay men. Eighteen months before, the AIDS caseload was only 41. Kramer criticizes those people who say this increase is statistically insignificant when compared with the vast number of homosexuals in the United States who do not have AIDS. The saturation rate of AIDS in gay men was high in New York City, where Kramer lived, with two cases reported per day; furthermore, the mortality rate began at 38 percent after diagnosis and rose to 86 percent at three years.[43]

Within the gay community, AIDS felt like a gay plague because it infected so many gay men in pockets like New York City and San Francisco and killed almost half within a year of diagnosis. One gay man in Los Angeles told his doctor in 1983, "I had sex with five or six people I know of who have the gay plague."[44] And Kramer captures the palpable threat the disease poses to the very existence of his community, like bubonic plague did centuries before him, when he proclaims, "in all the history of homosexuality we have never before been so close to death and extinction."[45]

The first made-for-TV-movie about AIDS in 1985, *An Early Frost*, captured this view of AIDS as a gay plague when the main character, Michael, is initially diagnosed. The movie was criticized by liberal voices that said it was not a realistic portrait of a middle-class family's ultimate acceptance of their gay son's diagnosis. More conservative views criticized the family's acceptance as an endorsement of homosexuality. In reality, it took Michael's sister and father the length of the movie to accept his AIDS diagnosis, and his father never really accepts his homosexuality, although he loves him and does not want him to die.[46]

Michael is a hard-working lawyer in a prominent Chicago law firm and naturally feels a bit run down, except that he has been having night sweats and fevers. When he finally goes to his doctor, he is hospitalized with PCP. Michael is amazed with the type of pneumonia that he has because it now means an AIDS diagnosis for him. And Michael has actually struggled with publically admitting his homosexuality. His partner, Peter, is often angry that he has not revealed their relationship to his family. Michael's reticence with his family in regard to his sexuality may feed his shock over his diagnosis now, but he is obviously aware of the perception of AIDS within the gay community. He asks his doctor upon discharge from the hospital, "How do I tell people I have the gay plague?"[47]

As the media increasingly covered AIDS as an illness that also affected non-gay men and as the number of cases began to increase overall, the "gay" in plague was shed. In early 1983, for instance, one journalist explains that AIDS "has now struck so many different groups," including intravenous drug users (IVDUs), their female partners, hemophiliacs, and Haitians.[48] The journalist does not specifically call these groups plague carriers but they are "struck" with the disease, a description that turns it into an affliction. Historically, an affliction suggests that the recipients deserve it in some way, as the Greeks did when Apollo "struck" them with his plague of arrows for stealing his priest's daughter. In fact, the journalist here distinguishes between the different groups of people "struck" by the illness who *do not* deserve it. Some of them are "innocent bystanders caught in the path of a new disease, [who] can make no behavioral decisions to minimize their risk."[49] The "innocent" include hemophiliacs, blood transfusion recipients, female partners of IVDUs, and babies. Everyone else with the disease (gays, IVDUs, and Haitians) was apparently *guilty* in contracting it; they must have deserved it. This innocent–guilty distinction ultimately will not work as we will see so-called "innocent bystanders" like Ryan White discriminated against for having the disease.

As the four risk groups—the 4Hs as they were popularly referred to at the time (homosexuals, heroin users, hemophiliacs, and Haitians)—were coalescing throughout 1983, descriptions of the disease as gay dimmed, but gay men were still the primary focus when it came to AIDS. An article in 1983 actually objected to the time when the disease was "derisively" called "the gay plague," but continues to point to a gay origin of the disease, which has the effect of isolating this group from everyone else. Gay men, the authors say, "still account for 72 percent" of the cases and "AIDS seems to be moving into the population at large."[50] The disease is still presented as moving *from* gay men *to* everyone else, when in reality 28 percent of everyone else had the disease alongside of these gay men. Furthermore, this article's presentation of AIDS as infecting non-gay populations only now in 1983, instead of acknowledging its presence in non-gays from the beginning, makes AIDS sound like a highly infectious disease beginning to run amuck.

Medical journals were not immune either to upholding a gay origin for the disease as the other risk groups were being established or to presenting

AIDS as a plague. The *Nursing Times* from England published "A 20th century Plague?" in August 1983. The subheading, "AIDS, originally thought to be an exclusively homosexual disease, is spreading its tentacles even wider," attempts to cast off the gay origin of the disease. The expression that it was "originally thought" to be a gay disease suggests that that view is now a mistaken one. But the picture on the first page of the article reveals two shirtless gay men dancing closely in "a gay disco in New York," as the caption reads, which keeps us thinking the origin of AIDS lies in gay men.[51] Like the *Newsweek* article a few months before this one, the focus shifts to other groups being infected with the disease and clearly it can no longer be "the gay plague" as the author implies. But it can be the "plague," as the title suggests, since it has spread to non-gay people and even non-American countries like England. AIDS is then aligned with bubonic plague in the Middle Ages by the time the article concludes. Travel in the twentieth century opens the possibility for "a worldwide epidemic of AIDS as terrifying as the Black Death of the thirteenth century."[52] We know that calling bubonic plague the "black death" in the Middle Ages is anachronistic since the phrase did not circulate until the sixteenth century in Sweden. We also know that the catastrophic second pandemic of bubonic disease occurred in the fourteenth and not in the thirteenth century. But myths also continued to abound regarding bubonic disease. Furthermore, there were only a couple of thousand cases of AIDS in America at this time and not the 50 million worldwide we would see by 2003.[53] Yet AIDS was being cradled by the centuries-long, global plague narrative.

Scourge, one of plague's synonyms, was also used at moments in 1983 to describe AIDS. Larry Kramer recognized that a percentage of AIDS cases was now occurring in non-gays but the disease had doubled in its incidence since his last eponymous AIDS statistics article written only six months before. Forty percent of those infected reside in New York City and the disease was "killing so many of my friends," as Kramer laments.[54] He holds the city's mayor and administration responsible for not funding programs that would assist in stemming its course, something that San Francisco's city government had done. He also criticizes the gay community's lack of support for GMHC's fund-raising events for AIDS. This lack of support provokes Kramer to ask for money from any international source in order "to investigate this *scourge*."[55] Past references to plague as "scourge" meant that it was some type of punishment. Kramer's usage of scourge for AIDS here also means that AIDS is a punishment in that it makes its victims needlessly suffer, but not in the traditional sense of a deserved punishment for some sin. After all, Kramer continues to be an outspoken and devoted voice for the rights of the gay community today.

Another newspaper article written during this year also referred to AIDS "as the scourge of a new disease" because it hurts those affected by it and not because they deserve it. This author, like Kramer, calls for AIDS victims to receive "more compassion" and "more resources" from the government.[56] Nonetheless, *scourge* is a culturally charged synonym for plague, and its employment in referring to AIDS, even by some liberal voices, taps into much older meanings of deserved punishment for some act considered sinful by a certain belief system. Labeling AIDS a plague, in spite of the intention behind the labeling, has the same effects in the late twentieth century as it did for bubonic disease in the medieval world and beyond.

Scientists suspected "the mysterious AIDS organism" was a virus prior to the 1984 American announcement of the viral discovery.[57] The mortality rate remained high with the number of cases rapidly increasing in major urban centers; even though collectively the number of AIDS cases across America remained low around 1,000 with 40 percent dead. But the lack of a cause for the disease in combination with rising cases and deaths provided "fertile ground for misinformation, superstitiousness, and magical thinking," as one Beth Israel physician in New York City pointed out in 1983.[58] Kramer's play *The Normal Heart* captures this type of thinking during these early years of the epidemic, the setting of his drama. This play dramatizes the founding of the GMHC and the obstacles the organization faced in the atmosphere of young men coming down with AIDS daily and dying quickly. Mickey, one of GMHC's cofounders, shares a seat in the waiting room of Dr. Emma Brookner's office early in the play when Bruce arrives with his sick partner. The doctor remembers caring for Bruce's former boyfriend who died a few weeks before. When Mickey hears this, he says, "it's like some sort of plague," because more and more people he knows are linked to this disease, the cause of which remains a mystery.[59] People in the Middle Ages certainly reached for the same term to explain bubonic disease. Modern medical theories by no means squelched magical thinking about infectious diseases.

Over a year later in Kramer's play, with GMHC up and running and still no cause of the disease discovered, Mickey continues to use the term *plague* to express his uneasiness with the unknowability surrounding AIDS. He anxiously asks other men at the GMHC office, "what if it's something out of the blue? The Great Plague of London was caused by polluted drinking water from a pump nobody noticed."[60] The London people of 1665 viewed their outbreak of bubonic disease as emerging "out of the blue," but with hindsight it seems that Dutch traders inadvertently carried the bacillus with them to English shores. These seventeenth-century Londoners thought God, comets, weather, and even rudimentary notions of microorganisms caused the outbreak, but polluted drinking water was not on the list. The polluted pump belongs to cholera's history from nineteenth-century London. Plague history continues to acquire its own myths here as AIDS joins its narrative.

Medieval views of plague as divine punishment for certain sins were not foreign either to the early 1980s when it came to AIDS. The gay community had notions of divine retribution in the form of AIDS for their own sexual behavior. The physician president of a gay caucus within the American Psychiatric Association in 1983 explained that gay men with AIDS "experienced a feeling of being punished for being gay."[61] Gay men at this time did not just imagine out of the blue that AIDS was a punishment for their sexual orientation. This idea is a strong legacy from plague narratives originating in the Middle Ages that were internalized in the late twentieth century by some very scared gay men. AIDS as divine punishment was also a circulating belief among the New Right and other conservatives at this time. Remember the New Orleans doctor mentioned earlier who said if AIDS was "God's punishment, it is not harsh enough."[62]

More specifically, this idea of deserving an illness because of one's behavior belongs to a time when discourse "for illness and life were [not yet] removed from the realm of moral and religious interpretation"—in other words, a time before the nineteenth century when illness was not yet embedded in scientific discourse.[63] Bubonic disease never really did achieve this status of being embedded substantively in scientific discourse and AIDS in the hands of more conservative people did not either. Cindy Patton explains, "AIDS is a particularly potent symbol" for the New Right "because it is evidence of sin" in their minds, and it is both a "sign and a punishment embodied in one of the groups targeted for political decimation long before AIDS."[64] AIDS is the manifestation of the consequences of a sexual orientation that is absolutely unacceptable for this politically and religious conservative group.

In this period, human causes of AIDS were also offered by writers as the disease was being constructed as a plague. Gay men were described as a cause without the assistance of divine intervention. In May 1982, one article reported that the CDC had been comparing the number of lifetime partners for gay men with AIDS to those without it. Men with AIDS had approximately 1,600 partners and those without it had 524 partners.[65] In addition, a prominent medical doctor the following year concluded that AIDS before 1981 was in "sporadic" form and therefore not identifiable, but now it had reached epidemic proportions, in large part, because of the "highly sexually active urban homosexual lifestyle."[66] The directly proportional relationship between the number of sexual partners and the incidence of AIDS in these articles makes gay men seem like they are the cause of it. Describing correlations between only gay male sex and the incidence of AIDS contributed to the milieu that, as Larry Kramer points out, "increasingly blamed [gay men] for AIDS, for the epidemic."[67]

Even after the discovery of the virus that caused AIDS, gay men were viewed by some as the disease's sole cause. Lockman's "guide" for "protecting" the public from AIDS advises Americans not to focus on the "innocents" who get AIDS but instead on "the homosexual nature of the AIDS menace" because "homosexuals and their biologically insane sex habits bear primary responsibility for bringing this plague upon us."[68] From this point of view, gay sexual orientation and acts cause this plague which non-gay people needlessly suffer from thanks to gay men. Kramer reminded Americans at this time, however, that gay men "are not the cause of AIDS but its victims."[69]

The other so-called "risk groups" for AIDS were victims of the disease as well, but often in subtle and not so subtle ways were described as its cause, especially those who did not achieve "innocent" status. By August 1982, as AIDS was being recognized in non-gay men, public health officials used plague discourse also to describe these people. The New York City health commissioner reported that "60 heterosexual" men and women who used drugs via "intravenous needles," "30 male and female immigrants from Haiti," and "some hemophiliacs" in addition to other "heterosexuals" who have received blood products have been "*afflicted*" with AIDS.[70] These people are not overtly blamed for having AIDS but the usage of this *plague* term implies some degree of punishment. Moreover, Susan Sontag poignantly argues, in her 1989 cultural piece on AIDS, that the creation of risk groups in general "revives the archaic idea of a tainted community that illness has judged."[71] Certain communities are only *made* to be "tainted" when some dominant social and political group, like the nineteenth-century British in Hong Kong, viewed and presented a less dominant group, like the Chinese there, as morally bankrupt and responsible for bubonic disease.

Hemophiliacs were never described as contracting AIDS because of some behavior on their part. They could not be blamed for the disease nor considered its cause. Their distinction from other risk groups lies exactly in their *inability* to control getting AIDS. An early 1983 article explains that "most of the nation's twenty thousand hemophiliacs have no choice about exposing themselves to possibly contaminated blood."[72] Hemophiliacs need the clotting factor VIII in order not to bleed to death, and it is made from multidonor plasma that carried the unknown AIDS virus at this time. This description of hemophiliacs' innocence in contracting AIDS implies that those risk groups who *have a choice* in exposing themselves to AIDS are indeed somehow responsible for getting the disease.

Gay men, according to this article, are even assigned blame for introducing AIDS into the IVDU population because "5 percent of the homosexual victims also shoot drugs."[73] IVDUs and homosexuals were viewed by many Americans in the early 1980s as having a choice in regard to their respective behaviors. Gays should simply choose to be straight and addicts should simply stop shooting drugs. In this line of thought, if one can choose not to be gay or shoot drugs, then one can avoid exposure to and transmission of this unknown AIDS bug. Suggesting certain behaviors are responsible for the spread of AIDS echoes accusations in the fourteenth century about the Jewish community's assumed behavior of poisoning wells that was believed to cause the spread of bubonic plague. *Yersinia pestis*, and not Jewish poisoning, caused bubonic disease and HIV causes AIDS. Having unprotected sex and using dirty needles potentially transmit the causative agent but not the actual act of having any kind of sex or shooting drugs.

Some writers in the early 1980s classified hemophiliacs, blood transfusion recipients, female partners of IVDUs, and babies as the "innocent bystanders" of the disease but Haitians did not make this list.[74] According to this "innocent/guilty" distinction, one may assume that Haitians must have engaged in some type of behavior that results in AIDS since they are not classified as "innocent." But according to American reports they did not. One of the first articles detailing Haitians with the disease claimed that out of the 34 cases of AIDS found in Haitian immigrants to the United States, 23 men who were asked about homosexuality denied it, and only one in 26 of these men admitted using intravenous drugs.[75] The reader is led to conclude that almost all of these Haitian AIDS cases were not gay or drug abusers. So what makes them an implied "guilty" risk group for AIDS? Haitians just might have become another source of AIDS *because* of their ethnicity, just as the Chinese were viewed by the British to be a source of bubonic plague.

Saidel Lane, M.D., the president of the Haitian Medical Association, saw a problem with the way the questions were posed by American doctors to these Haitian immigrants with AIDS. Dr. Lane said that just expecting a "yes or no answer" for whether or not the patient is gay or an IVDU usually results in "a *no* answer because homosexuality or even IV drug use is a tough subject to accept in Haitians."[76] It seems that these American doctors did not understand the particular cultural values that prevented Haitians from admitting these behaviors. It was also no wonder that Haitian immigrants denied these behaviors considering that Americans who admitted to them were blamed for getting this disease that was blossoming into a full-blown plague in the psyche of our society.

The scientifically proven and most rational cause of AIDS was the discovery of the human immunodeficiency virus. Work began on identifying the virus soon after the persistent appearance of AIDS in France and the United States. Scientists from both countries had promising causative microbes.

Luc Montagnier, M.D., at the Pasteur Institute in Paris discovered LAV (lymphadenopathy-associated virus) in 1983 and antibodies from several infected patients were isolated there. Robert Gallo, M.D., an American scientist at the National Cancer Institute, also isolated HTLV-III (human T-lymphotropic virus type three) that at first appeared to be a different virus from the French one. U.S. secretary of Health and Human Services Margaret Heckler announced the discovery of Dr. Gallo's virus on April 23, 1984, but only facilely acknowledged the French discovery. In 2008, however, the Nobel Prize in Medicine was solely granted to Dr. Montagnier, and not to Dr. Gallo, for the discovery of HIV.

By 1985 when antibody testing became widely available for the AIDS virus—officially named HIV then in order to neutrally acknowledge the discovery made by both AIDS scientists—AIDS continued to be described as a plague. The discovery of *Yersinia pestis* as the causative agent of bubonic, pneumonic, and septicemic disease also did not stop the British in Hong Kong, Americans in San Francisco, and diverse writers throughout the twentieth century from referring to the disease as plague, either. As a matter of fact, with almost 7,000 total AIDS cases reported in the United States, as 1985 opened, in a population of more than 200 million people and the viral cause identified, AIDS was now called "The New Plague" by major newspapers.[77] And a *Life* magazine article's title warned, "Now No One Is Safe from AIDS," as if 7 million instead of 7,000 cases had been reported.[78] AIDS apparently now qualified as "the new plague" because the virus "will kill man, woman, or child if a sufficient dose gets into the bloodstream."[79] The potentially ubiquitous nature of viral infection makes AIDS a plague here. Yet this presentation of widespread viral transmission did not render the risk groups for AIDS obsolete, and interestingly heterosexuals were cocooned from joining them. One journalist reiterates the percentages of the different groups with AIDS and stresses that "AIDS is transmitted very rarely through heterosexual sex."[80] Obviously there was still some misunderstanding about how *any* type of *unprotected* sexual act can potentially transmit the virus. But misunderstandings are essential to plague-making.

Sontag insightfully offered that " 'plague' is the principal metaphor by which the AIDS epidemic is understood."[81] AIDS, like bubonic disease, is feared by so many people and this is the common variable, as Sontag sees it, which facilitates the usage of the metaphor for any feared disease. Yet AIDS may have been so feared to begin with, and still is, because of this cultural making of it as a plague.

Classic reactions to plague, such as fear and scapegoating, occurred with the emergence of AIDS as it was being constructed as a plague in newspaper articles, scientific journals, movies, and plays. *An Early Frost* captures the fear of contagion in the more private realm of interpersonal relations. When Michael returns home to his apartment with Peter after his initial hospitalization, Peter will not share his cup like he always had done, and their close set of friends who were coming to dinner cancelled their visit. Michael asks Peter, "Are they afraid they will get AIDS from eating pasta?"[82] People were. My own parents in Pennsylvania, who always supported my decision to work with AIDS patients, asked me quite innocently after I began my tenure on the AIDS unit, "Do we need to buy a separate set of silverware for you to use at dinner when you come home again?" And I was only *working* with AIDS patients.

Michael's sister, Susan, is quite happy in the movie when her brother tells her that he told their parents he was gay, but having AIDS was another story. Susan tells Michael she hopes he does not have the disease because of the "terrible stories" she hears about it. When Michael admits his diagnosis to her, she will not let him touch her son. She also views his AIDS as a particular threat to her unborn baby. Susan justifies her distance from Michael because she feels that she "needs to think about my family."[83] Beliefs that everyone was vulnerable to this disease through casual contact were prevalent as the disease gained plague status. Susan does hug Michael good-bye at the end of the movie when he returns to Chicago, but we are not convinced that her extreme fear of catching AIDS casually has abated. It seems more likely that her love for her brother temporarily overrides this fear.

During the early 1980s, the United States also experienced a very public fear of casual contact contagion with AIDS. In 1983 with AIDS cases surpassing 200 in San Francisco, landlords were evicting their tenants with AIDS, as if the walls of the apartments were contaminated from their presence.[84] Granted the viral cause of AIDS was not known at this time, but there was not one single case reported from casual contact. Police officers in San Francisco were also quite fearful of any contact with AIDS patients as they wore masks and gloves when they were even near "a suspected" one, which of course meant anyone police officers thought was gay. The deputy police chief there explained how "we have a large homosexual population" and "the officers were concerned they could bring the bug home" and their whole family could get AIDS.[85] In the Middle Ages, bubonic plague was thought to be transmitted by just looking at infected victims. In the minds of many late-twentieth-century San Franciscans, close proximity to someone who was merely suspected of being gay meant a possible transmission of AIDS.

Gay men were not the only source of fear, so were infected schoolchildren and blood banks. A newspaper article's title in December 1985 recognizes that "Hysteria Is behind the Drive to Bar AIDS Victims from Schools."[86]

New Jersey residents did not want children who were even suspected of having AIDS to attend public schools. At the same time, another article's title reads, "AIDS Fears Cut Blood Donations."[87] The Long Island Blood Services reported this decrease in blood donations because people feared contracting the AIDS virus from just donating blood. Certainly fears about contracting AIDS from receiving a blood transfusion persisted and were less a result of AIDS' presentation as a plague by writers. It was a fact that prior to the HIV antibody test, some people received infected blood. But hysteria about schoolchildren passing the virus on to others through play at recess or by sitting next to someone in the classroom and about *just donating* blood when sterile needles are used without contact with anyone else's blood has been produced as a result of the growing plague mentality surrounding AIDS. And unlike bubonic disease, AIDS was never transmitted casually.

This fear of AIDS did not bypass the medical community, either. Medical doctors prior to 1981 were quite secure in knowing that infectious diseases, such as bubonic disease, tuberculosis, and smallpox were treatable with antibiotics and vaccines. Herzlich and Pierret explain that in France this triumphant view of infectious diseases belongs to the "victories of medicine" discourse that we certainly experienced here in America, as well.[88] An October 1984 article on AIDS explains that those of us in "privileged" countries—meaning developed countries with available medicines that effectively treat illnesses—usually do not live with the threat of "deadly, incurable infectious diseases," nor do we "live in fear of plague."[89]

When AIDS unexpectedly and officially arrived in the United States in 1981, many health-care professionals found themselves living with this fear of plague. One journalist notes that although doctors in particular knew that AIDS could not be transmitted by touch, they still wore gowns, masks, and gloves just to talk with patients. This way overly cautious protective garb worn when not performing a risky procedure, such as a bone marrow biopsy or spinal tap, may indicate medical doctors' response "to the ancient fear of contagion."[90] In other words, they were projecting fears about diseases like so-called bubonic plague "when medicine had less power over microbes" onto AIDS when it emerged.[91] Doctors were not the only medical personnel projecting these fears. A nurse who was floated to my unit one evening after one of our regular nurses called in sick refused to enter any of the patients' rooms. I asked her how she would take care of her assigned patients and she replied, "I don't know, but I won't touch them."

These fears in conjunction with the isolated risk groups for AIDS led to a fair amount of scapegoating of people with AIDS. When Ryan White, the 13-year-old Indiana hemophiliac, developed AIDS in 1984, it did not take long before his high school discovered his diagnosis. In spite of the health commissioner there advising Ryan's principal to allow him to attend school as long as he was not too ill, which he was not at the time, the school board voted to bar him from school, and 50 teachers vowed they would not have him in their classrooms. When Ryan was legally allowed to return to school in early 1986, he had to agree to use disposable cutlery and plates in the cafeteria, and he could not use public drinking fountains or bathrooms. But this was not enough. After only one day back at school, a parents' group threatened to sue the school board if Ryan was allowed to continue attending classes. Even though Americans knew by 1984 that HIV caused AIDS and it was not transmitted by sitting next to someone in a classroom, or by using the same washed silverware, or by drinking from the same fountain, Ryan White became the pariah of his community.

More discrimination followed after this parents' group forced Ryan back into the seclusion of his home. He was vilified by other children with deroga-tory adjectives usually reserved for gay men. They called him "fag" as beer cans and garbage were hurled on his front lawn. Even when he was again allowed to return to school, other children wrote "faggot" and "queer" on his folders.[92] The culturally assigned gay nature of AIDS not only stuck but was reserved for expressing the most vehement hatred for an AIDS victim. The feigned distinction between "innocent" and "guilty" risk groups for AIDS did not preclude the discrimination experienced by all of them.

In the eyes of many medical doctors, Haitians were presumably like hemophiliacs in terms of having no defining behavior that led to contract-ing AIDS, and also they were the victims of scapegoating. Haitians, unlike hemophiliacs, however, were not touted as an "innocent" risk group and their ethnicity explains their risk and the resultant discrimination they faced. A brief look at U.S.-Haiti relations will provide some insight into how Haitians became perceived plague carriers during the early years of the AIDS epidemic. In the early 1960s, Haiti was, to a degree, dominated economically by the United States. Our country turned Haiti into "a low-wage, export-friendly economy that provided profitable business opportunities for U.S. investors."[93] Over the next few decades, U.S. investment opportunities grew in this small country while economic opportunities for Haitian workers did not. By the 1980s, Haiti was ranked among the top ten nations that provided America with goods such as baseballs, toys, and clothing. Haitians were an easy target of blame for AIDS by its economic colonizer, the United States, when some of them developed the disease just as the Chinese with bubonic plague were in the eyes of their British colonizers. The threat of American profits decreasing in Haiti and the threat of a paucity of cheap imported goods from there might have provoked a certain degree of American dis-dain for potential economic losses to be projected onto Haitians with AIDS.

This disease in Haitians potentially threatened U.S. economic progress in our own country, especially if too many of them got it, just as bubonic disease among Chinese in Hong Kong threatened Great Britain's global progress.

In addition, American ignorance about Haitian cultural beliefs and customs led to a facile assignment of them as a "guilty" risk group for AIDS that resulted in scapegoating them. An American doctor in 1983 stressed that Haitians "are involved in voodoo and spiritualism," which could play a role in the transmission of AIDS.[94] But this doctor, and the journalist writing about him, do not discuss Haitian religious practices, such as sacrificial ceremonies for certain spirits, in order to specifically explore a potential transmission of the disease. Proposing any unexplained association between Haitian voodoo and the transmission of AIDS perpetuates magical thinking about this ethnic group and the disease.

Haitians living in the United States in the early 1980s certainly experienced discrimination as a result of this forged association. According to one journalist, Haitians here felt like they had "become victims of a new outbreak of social discrimination" because "they have been labeled carriers of a deadly disease." In this year, Haitians reported job losses and an inability to sell their homes in the United States, and those in Haiti reported a 20 percent fall in tourism from the previous year.[95]

In reality by mid-1983, only 102 of the 1,922 nationally reported AIDS cases occurred in Haitians. New York City health officials actually removed them as an AIDS risk group at this time because only 31 of the 877 cases there were Haitians and they felt this "small number" did not justify "stigmatizing" them.[96] Unfortunately, the CDC did not remove Haitians as a risk group until May 1985 when they were relegated into the "other/unknown" risk category. Guarded discrimination ensued on some level with the CDC's recommendation that Haitian entrants to the United States refrain from donating blood or plasma along with "sexually active homosexual/bisexual men with multiple partners," IVDUs, and hemophiliacs. Their rationale was that 5 percent of Haitian-Americans who were tested as controls for HIV antibodies were found to be HIV positive.[97] Haitians' new classification as "other/unknown" kept them in a risk group still based solely on their ethnic "otherness."

But not surprisingly, gay men were the primary scapegoats for AIDS. A certain degree of hatred, or even misunderstanding, of the gay community coupled with fear of contracting the disease resulted in varying degrees of discrimination. One doctor in 1983 described how gay men feared "the fate of another group of diseased individuals—lepers."[98] Lepers usually have been shunned by their societies and sometimes even blamed for inexplicable events like the contamination of the water supply in Languedoc, France in the early fourteenth century.

Unfortunately, these fears in the gay male community came to fruition during these early years of the AIDS epidemic. In June 1983, for example, a New York City hospital patient with AIDS paid a good amount of money for his hospital room but did not receive any housekeeping services during his stay.[99] He even had to clean his own bathroom. On the AIDS unit I worked on, even in the late 1980s we were often hard-pressed to get housekeepers to enter any of our patients' rooms as they trembled at the thought of coming into contact with any surface touched by our patients. The nursing staff usually cleaned up any spills in the rooms. The patient who performed his own housekeeping services also faced more discrimination when his partner flew him back to Arizona to be with his mother. When he died, the hospital staff wrapped sheets around him and placed him in a plastic bag instead of performing routine postmortem care. His undertaker then poured embalming fluid over the sheets instead of in his veins before placing his body in the casket.[100]

Larry Kramer's character Bruce in *The Normal Heart* echoes this scenario as he describes the awful treatment experienced by his dead partner. Bruce also took his dying partner back to Phoenix to be with his mother. When he died there, the doctors would not examine him nor place a cause of death on his death certificate. Consequently, undertakers would not retrieve the body at the hospital, and the hospital orderlies placed him "in a heavy-duty GLAD bag" for Bruce and his partner's mother to carry out of the hospital.[101] An undertaker was finally found to perform the cremation. Many of our patients' families had incredibly difficult times finding undertakers to prepare the bodies of their loved ones when AIDS appeared as the cause of death on their death certificates.

By 1986, acts of discrimination became even more public. In San Francisco as a gay man waited for his roommate at a supermarket, a young man and woman spewed venomous comments at him such as "we should kill you first because you're gonna give us AIDS."[102] This accusation is most telling for the success of AIDS' construction as a plague. These young people thought they could get the disease from simply being near someone they believed was gay. When more people arrived, the man's roommate was pulled out of the car by them and beaten. Three men in Brooklyn at this time also honed in on a gay man walking to the store in the morning. While beating him, they screamed, "Faggot! You faggots give us AIDS."[103] Gay men were certainly suffering from the societal construction of them as the principal plague vector.

Classic reactions to plague other than fear and scapegoating were particularly experienced by gay men during these early years of the epidemic. Despair was certainly expected as many gay men became ill and died from the disease. Nearing the end of 1985, the CDC reported that 8,241 of the 13, 061 AIDS cases since 1981 were gay or bisexual men—that is 63 percent of the AIDS burden was carried by them.[104] In major cities, like New York, funerals became the latest social event for members and affiliates of the gay community. Andrew Holleran's short story, *Friends at Evening* focuses on a group of gay male friends on their way to Louis' funeral. Mr. Lark describes Louis' illness and his death to Ned. When Ned asks if this disease will ever stop, Mr. Lark's stark response is diametrically opposed to his surname: "I think we're all going to die."[105] Hope was hard to sustain at this time.

There is a form of hope, however, in the reaction of anger to AIDS, especially anger channeled into political action. Anger has not been a prevalent reaction to plague in the past, except maybe in that Chinese grocer in San Francisco who filed a lawsuit against the city when his neighboring white business owners were not subjected to the quarantine like his shop was during the plague outbreak there. An awareness of discrimination for being a plague carrier seemed to provoke an angry reaction in these victims. Many of Kramer's essays contain angry reactions to AIDS that grow throughout this period culminating in the founding of ACT UP (AIDS Coalition to Unleash Power). Kramer, for instance, intended for his groundbreaking essay, "1,112 and Counting," to "rouse [readers] to anger, fury, rage, and action" in order to overturn what he saw was becoming institutionalized discrimination against AIDS victims.[106] Kramer saw anger as the motivator for propelling the CDC into action for tracking how the disease is spread, for doctors to offer more treatment options unduly bogged down in bureaucracy, for hospital staff to be educated about AIDS, and for the government to approve disability benefits for AIDS patients. He ultimately called for "demonstrations of civil disobedience" in order to begin the path of resolving these discriminatory issues.[107]

Less emotionally charged reactions to AIDS were also witnessed during the first few years of the disease's appearance. These reactions remind us why AIDS was not a plague, even though the cultural current tended to drown this antiplague mentality. This rationality we have seen in other centuries dealing with diseases created as plagues, such as in early twentieth-century San Francisco catching rats and building cement buildings in order to stem bubonic disease there. Though *An Early Frost* appeared early in the epidemic, and in spite of contributing to views of AIDS as a plague, the movie also presents more rational responses that represent an antiplague mentality. Michael's grandmother remembers how people treated her husband like a leper because of his cancer diagnosis. She tells Michael that people stayed away from him and acted as if they could contract the disease from the air. Her gesture of kissing Michael rejects paranoiac fears of casual contagion with the virus like we see in his sister, Susan. When Michael pulls away from his grandmother as she attempts to kiss him, she retorts, "it's a disease, not a disgrace."[108] Whenever AIDS is viewed as a plague it is a "disgrace," and when it is viewed rationally, it is simply a disease.

In early 1986, a journalist recognized that "a plague mentality" distorted rational thought when it came to the discriminatory treatment experienced by children with AIDS.[109] The article, actually written by a Republican in the New Jersey State Senate, argues that because of what we know about the viral transmission of HIV, it is ridiculous to fear children with AIDS in public schools. The author debunks the by now popular notion that AIDS is a highly infectious disease by reminding his readers that "AIDS is not tuberculosis, measles or the flu."[110] He attributes parents' and school boards' lack of faith in the medical community's issued facts on AIDS transmission to "a plague mentality [that] has taken over."[111] This mentality developed during the first five years of AIDS' appearance and growth as the disease was *made* a plague.

CHAPTER 7

Solidifying Plague (1987–1989)

I reported on duty for my first shift on the AIDS unit during the frigid Thanksgiving week of 1987. The unit had only eight beds at the time but they were never empty for long. The only two requirements for admission to this elite club were a diagnosis of full-blown AIDS and an awareness of it. We did not want anyone surprised as we openly discussed the myriad issues surrounding the illness with all of our patients; at least half of them were housed in a four-bedded room. I was struck by Kimberly, the lone female there. Years later on our unit, this gender disparity would balance itself out, but for now, like the rest of America in 1987, I primarily viewed AIDS as a gay male disease. After all, I had only cared for these men with the disease until this point.

Kimberly was tough, polite, and in constant need of a cigarette. "Could you do me a favor?" she would always ask the nursing staff who reentered her room whether after only ten minutes or one hour. "Can I have a cigarette?" Her first visit to our unit was for PCP, but in a few months after her next bout she experienced a seizure that signaled her *Toxoplasmosis gondii*—this diagnosis made our unit her permanent residence. After her open brain biopsy to diagnose this protozoan parasite that infects the brain of immunocompromised patients, her quick wit dissipated but she retained her pleasant demeanor and her appetite for cigarettes.

Kimberly talked about her daughter from time to time. When we asked her if we could call her before the brain surgery she said, "Don't bother. She stopped bothering with me a long time ago." Her daughter had been raised by Kimberly's mother when heroin lured Kimberly away from everyone she loved. When we asked Kimberly if her daughter knew that she was sick, she replied, "Yeah. She said I deserve it." We never met Kimberly's daughter or mother in all the months she stayed with us. They neglected her like many families of plague victims had done in past centuries. We were it for her as she lay dying on our unit.

These next few years in the AIDS epidemic were significant foremost for the unusually rational report on AIDS issued by our quite religiously and politically conservative surgeon general, C. Everett Koop, and for the irrational disconnect that persisted in the plague-making of AIDS. The *Surgeon General's Report on Acquired Immune Deficiency Syndrome* was published on October 22, 1986, and it was not what conservatives expected inside or outside President Ronald Reagan's administration.[1] Koop, after all, was a Christian fundamentalist and no one expected him to openly discuss sexual intercourse practices that could spread HIV, such as "penis-vagina, penis-rectum, and mouth-rectum" intercourse.[2] Yet Dr. Koop is a physician, a professional who is supposed to adhere to an objective approach to the human body under study. Koop's *Report* had the intent of destigmatizing or deplaguing the first five years of the AIDS epidemic. In it he stresses that AIDS cannot be contracted through casual contact, a perception that arose in American minds as AIDS gained plague status. He admits that the disease is certainly "an infectious disease, but not spread like common cold or measles."[3] He also openly discusses condom usage to decrease the spread of HIV. He also addresses the hysteria over HIV negative children attending school with those who were positive by reiterating that no AIDS cases have resulted from casual contact.[4]

Although Koop does not overtly recognize that AIDS had been made into a plague like I do, he certainly recognizes discriminatory attitudes toward people with AIDS and advocates overturning them. He mentions that many Americans have not exhibited any sympathy for people with the disease and in fact think that they "deserve" it. Koop makes it clear that this type of blaming mind frame prevents us from "preserving our humanity."[5] His covert criticism of the discriminators of AIDS victims, who viewed the disease as a moral as opposed to a physical illness, exemplified a rational response to an epidemic that had been irrationally handled by members of Koop's own medical and religious communities.

Koop was not alone during this time in his attempts to approach AIDS in this manner. The scientist Stephen Jay Gould wrote an editorial for *The New York Times* in April 1987 titled "The Terrifying Normalcy of AIDS," and the "terrifying" in his title refers to how "normal" AIDS is when looked at from a scientific perspective. Gould articulates that the disease's emergence is natural and we need to address it, not by ignoring its potential spread to all groups of people, but by treating it like any other disease. AIDS is not, he says, "an irrational or diabolical plague with a moral meaning."[6]

In another editorial released one month after Gould's, Burton Levine dismissed any similarities between AIDS and plague. Levine primarily will not grant AIDS plague status because it has not killed as many people as bubonic disease did during its most severe outbreaks like we saw in the fourteenth century. Koop revealed approximately 25,000 cases of known AIDS, with half of those infected dead near the end of 1986, and we remember how many people died from bubonic disease in any given European country alone within a few short years in the mid-fourteenth century.[7] Levine reminds his readers that "AIDS would have had to kill 79 million Americans from 1981 to 1985" in order to "equal" the so-called plague's toll. The statistical disparity between plague and AIDS, however, is not the only reason Levine will not grant AIDS plague status. He notices that when AIDS is compared to the medieval plague, it "increases panic" by conjuring up "those images" of plague and "attaching them" to AIDS.[8]

These rational voices unfortunately were muffled by those who contributed to solidifying AIDS' plague status even more. Fictional works on AIDS continued to refer to it as plague. Writers of fiction, after all, engage with and work out imaginatively—whether consciously or not—the fears, hopes, and desires circulating in the society in which they live. And there were plenty of emotions surrounding AIDS in 1980s America to engage with and work out. Edmund White's 1986 short story, "An Oracle," for instance, focuses on a character named Roy who lost his partner George to AIDS about a year before the story begins. When Roy's friend arranges a trip to Crete for him, his attention quickly turns to a young male prostitute, Marco, whom he pays for sex nightly. Roy reflects on how amazing it is in Crete to achieve physical intimacy, something he has missed in "his plagued city" of New York. Being so far away from home, Roy wonders whether or not Marco has even heard of "our deadly disease." The profound losses in the gay male community of New York City are captured here in Roy's descriptions of home in America.[9]

But we tend to expect nonfictional genres, such as journalism, to present AIDS in less imaginative ways. During this period, newspaper articles, magazines, medical journals, and nonfictional books continued to describe AIDS as a plague. An article in *The New York Times* written in early 1987 actually claimed that "AIDS may dwarf the plague," in addition to small pox and typhoid epidemics.[10] The 25,000 cases of AIDS at the time in America could not even compare to the millions of smallpox cases in the twentieth century, nor to the hundreds of thousands of typhoid cases in the French army during Napoleon's invasion of Russia in the early nineteenth century, let alone to the annihilation of populations across the globe from bubonic disease in the Middle Ages and beyond. AIDS was far from "dwarfing" so-called plague, smallpox, and typhoid in 1987.

In his book critiquing journalists and the media for initially not covering AIDS and then for turning the reporting into drama, James Kinsella would have classified this article on AIDS "dwarfing" the plague as representative of the "sensationalistic" coverage of the epidemic that began in the mid-1980s.[11] This "sensationalism" certainly contributed to the view that AIDS was a plague and in turn produced even more panic surrounding the mention of the disease. As valuable as Kinsella's book is for this type of critique, his own title, *Covering the Plague: AIDS and the American Media*, does not assist in desensationalizing the disease.

Medical journals tended to be less hyperbolic about AIDS than newspaper articles, but the disease was still described as a plague during this time. Dr. Robert Gallo, the erstwhile co-discoverer of HIV, in 1987 begins his article "The AIDS Virus" by describing it as "a modern plague," which he qualifies by discussing the disease's "pandemic" status.[12] In epidemiological terms, a pandemic simply means a disease that has infected people throughout the world without specifically referring to the number of people infected or the nature of the disease. Pandemic does not translate as plague. Gallo's description of the action of the virus he claims to have discovered is colorful as well, which has the effect of exaggerating its properties and stimulating emotions of panic. "The virus *bursts* into action," he tells us, and "reproduces itself so *furiously*" in its quest to obliterate T4 lymphocytes, its main target in the immune system.[13]

Gallo also uses plague discourse in his first article published with Dr. Luc Montagnier in October 1988. As these scientists turn to discussing possible treatments for AIDS after describing how the virus works and how it might have emerged in Africa, they ask, "What weapons are available against this *scourge*?"[14] They do not imply that scourge is any kind of deserved punishment, but the connotation of this *plague* synonym attached to AIDS has cultural consequences. It perpetuates viewing AIDS as a plague in readers of *Scientific American*, many of whom were in the medical community caring for AIDS patients.

The U.S. president's silence on AIDS during the first six years of the epidemic certainly did not help in steering the public away from viewing it as a plague and toward viewing it as just another infectious disease that needed to be stopped quickly. It is not surprising to read an article announcing in May 1987, before President Ronald Reagan addressed the AIDS crisis in America, that "we live in a time of plague such as has never been visited on our nation."[15] Of course the 1918 influenza pandemic killed more than half a million Americans in one year, which seems to qualify more as a plague than AIDS does, if plague is defined as a highly infectious disease with a high mortality rate. AIDS had not killed anywhere close to even 100,000 people at this time.

When Reagan finally uttered the word "AIDS" during the Third International AIDS Conference, more than 36,000 Americans had been diagnosed with AIDS, with almost 21,000 dead from it.[16] These statistics do not suggest that AIDS was as infectious or as lethal as the 1918 flu, rather that there were a substantial number of people contracting and dying from this syndrome announced by the CDC six years before Reagan acknowledged it. The president's silence facilitated misconceptions about AIDS as a plague because he never addressed the nature of the disease and the means of transmission adequately. During this first speech on AIDS on May 31, 1987, Reagan did not mention the toll of the disease on the gay community, and his main focus was on testing for HIV in an effort to stop its spread as opposed to focusing on safe sex education and clean needle usage.[17] Mention of his surgeon general's *Report* on AIDS issued only seven months before also was woefully missing from the speech.

In essence, Reagan's speech endorsed the discrimination of AIDS patients even more, especially with its hints of mandatory HIV testing without confidentiality. The New Right's influence was evident in the president's advocacy of testing instead of educating people about unsafe sexual practices and drug use that could transmit the virus. Gay men feared the development of quarantine camps after hearing Reagan speak. Anyone who had ever engaged in a behavior that could have resulted in contracting HIV also feared getting tested for it. No one wanted to be denied jobs, health care, or life insurance if discovered to be HIV positive. After all, Haitians lost jobs and homes in America just because they were designated as a risk group for AIDS by the CDC.

A few months after Reagan's speech, *Newsweek* released a photo "journal of a single plague year," its feature article for the August 1987 edition.[18] The magazine's cover is wall-to-wall photos of people from diverse age groups, ethnicities, and genders who are all "the face of AIDS."[19] During this "plague" year, "302 men, women, and children" captured in the photos died; they are among the annual total casualty of four thousand.[20] Now the disease knew no boundaries, making it seem like it really was a plague, as the article would have us believe. *Newsweek's* "journal of a plague year" certainly takes us back to Daniel Defoe's *A Journal of the Plague Year* a few centuries ago and assists in securing the position of AIDS in the global plague narrative once again.

In spite of the viral cause of AIDS being discovered in 1984, divine and human ones continued to be offered for this epidemic just as they were after the bacterial discovery of bubonic disease in the late nineteenth century. One theologian, in the late 1980s, explores, from a Catholic perspective, whether or not AIDS is "divine judgment" for sins.[21] Gilbert Meilaender initially contemplates whether or not all illnesses are incurred by chance or determined by some specific factor. He uses the behavior of smoking cigarettes often resulting in lung cancer as support for illnesses not being random. He extends this rationale to support a behavioral etiology of AIDS. He sees that not all cases of lung cancer come from smoking and not all cases of AIDS come from sexual promiscuity or drug abuse, but enough do to qualify these behaviors as causative factors of illness incurred ultimately because of divine judgment.

Meilaender attempts to get some "critical distance" from this weighty issue of behavior causing illness, and ironically turns to Defoe's *Journal of the Plague Year* for textual and historical support of his argument.[22] Defoe's journal, however, is a fictional account of a factual event. Meilaender discusses Defoe's episode of the taverners who mock the mourning man and later die from the plague presumably because they were punished by God with the disease for their taunting behavior. Meilaender concludes that Defoe "believes that sin brings divine punishment" in the form of plague. Defoe's sinning taverners ultimately support his view that "casual sexual contact or promiscuity," behaviors that qualify as sins for Christians, invite divine punishment in the form of AIDS.[23] Although Meilaender's slim booklet probably did not reach a wide audience, just as Lawrence Lockman's *Guide* for protecting the public from the plague of AIDS did not, it is notable for its persistent medieval view of what constitutes a sin, for using sin as an explanation for divine causes of diseases, and for how fragile the philosophical and theological foundation of this argument really is. After all, Meilaender's support for his position is a fictional account written a century after the bubonic disease outbreak in seventeenth-century London. Nonetheless, this treatise was probably read by enough fellow Christians, and it contributed to forging the lineage between so-called plagues of earlier centuries and AIDS in the late twentieth century.

Divine causes of AIDS were, however, proposed by people at this time who reached a wider audience. The voice of the New Right, the Moral Majority, offered them. Televangelist Jerry Falwell said at this time that "AIDS is the wrath of God upon homosexuals."[24] Pat Buchanan, Reagan's communication director, said mockingly in May 1983 that "the poor homosexuals—they have declared war upon nature, and now nature is exacting an awful retribution."[25] This ultraconservative view positions homosexuality against Nature de facto. The usage of "nature" by Buchanan harkens back to medieval notions of a natural order being ordained by God. The medieval world viewed peasants as violating the natural social order when they demanded more wages for their labor, and this violation was proposed by writers then as being responsible for plague's arrival.

In this pronouncement, Buchanan implies that twentieth-century homosexuality violates the natural order of sexual relations between a man and a woman, and this violation incurs divine retribution in the form of AIDS. According to this view, plague also serves as a corrective for a sexual orientation that violates Buchanan's conservative belief system. I mention Buchanan's explanation of AIDS as divine punishment from 1983 not only because his description *turns* the disease into a plague but also because this statement reached a lot of people when Randy Shilts quoted it in 1987 in *And the Band Played On.*

Proposing human causes for AIDS persisted in this period, as well. The risk groups established for AIDS earlier in the decade were still maintained by the medical establishment and mainstream media that in essence locked these people into being viewed as the only actual or potential carriers of AIDS. Instead of drawing attention to *how* HIV was transmitted, as Dr. Koop did in his *Report* when he discussed the viral transmission in different bodily fluids during different sexual activities, the CDC continued to pay attention to *who* was transmitting HIV in its final yearly tally of AIDS cases in December 1986. This edition of the *MMWR* says that "97 percent of all adult AIDS patients can be placed in groups," with homosexuals and bisexuals comprising 66 percent of the cases and heterosexual IVDUs holding 17 percent. The CDC's intent was to discern "a possible *means* of disease acquisition" by focusing on *who* has the disease.[26] But we already knew the *means* from Koop's *Report* published a few months before this one.

A *New York Times* article in early 1987 reinforces the CDC's "groups" instead of Koop's *means* of HIV transmission by claiming "there is no clear evidence that AIDS in the United States has yet spread beyond the known risk groups, notably homosexuals and drug addicts."[27] This continued focus on *who* gets AIDS stigmatizes certain behaviors instead of highlighting *how* the virus is transmitted during sexual acts and drug use. In effect, these groups carry the blame for spreading AIDS and everyone outside of these groups can believe they are safe from the disease, a dangerous misconception that provided non-gays and non-IVDUs with the illusion that their own unprotected intimate behavior was *naturally* safe.

A focus on another sexual group as an AIDS carrier emerged in the later 1980s, and this group was surrounded by plague discourse in one of the first *New York Times* articles introducing its behavior as a risk for AIDS. The bisexual man is the "AIDS Specter for Women," an April 1987 title tells us. This man, who is "cloaked in myth and his own secretiveness, has become the *bogeyman* of the late 1980s." He is presented as specifically haunting straight women by hiding his sexuality while harboring the deadly virus.[28]

This new AIDS threat became a palpable reality a few years later when New York City native Alison Gertz revealed that she contracted AIDS from a sexual encounter with a man in the early 1980s whom she later discovered was bisexual and died from AIDS. Gertz never really blamed this man during her public educational talks to young people advocating safe sex for everyone, regardless of sexual orientation. But by the time she publically conveyed the irrelevancy of *who* one has sex with, it was too late for bisexual men to be exonerated as plague carriers.[29]

The construction of the bisexual man as the new bogeyman for AIDS also did nothing for making many of these men feel comfortable enough to admit their sexuality to themselves, let alone to anyone else; this denial often led to unsafe sexual practices. A psychologist in New Jersey who counseled gays and bisexuals explained that many bisexual men would not practice safe sex "because that would be an admission that it is high-risk, homosexual behavior." Even bisexual men in San Francisco who did admit their sexual practices "feared they will become scapegoated as carriers of the plague."[30] As we have seen, being gay or practicing sexual acts considered to be gay in the 1980s meant being a potential or actual plague carrier. This perception will contribute to the spread of AIDS in the African American community over the next two decades because "the down low" man could no sooner admit his sexual practices either without risking severe discrimination.

Some in the gay male community in the late 1980s, not surprisingly, began to internalize society's view of them as the cause of AIDS by blaming themselves. Andrew Holleran explores why gay men are not angrier at the U.S. government's inaction in responding to AIDS in his 1988 piece, "The Absence of Anger." He explains that many gay men actually do not even accept their own sexuality and are not aware of their own "self-hatred" produced as a result of this denial. Holleran matter-of-factly refers to AIDS as the "plague" here because it affected so many in his community, and he observes that the disease's prevalence had "gay men in doctors' offices all over Manhattan weeping over their pasts." Some of them even echoed Pat Buchanan in regretting their homosexuality because *it* was the cause of having AIDS—or so they thought.[31]

Paul Monette shares Holleran's insights about gay male self-loathing resulting in self-blame for having AIDS in his 1988 memoir, *Borrowed Time*. As Monette begins to chronicle how he and Roger, his partner and soul mate, realized that Roger was ill, he not only facilely refers to AIDS as a "plague," but blames himself for giving it to Roger. "None of this would be happening if I'd never had sex with strangers," he thinks. Of course, he also knows that Roger could have contracted AIDS from one of his own unprotected, previous sexual encounters but he still feels guilty. Paul also realizes that "all the self-hating years in the closet" contributed to this self-blame now for having AIDS.[32] Gay men viewing themselves as the cause of AIDS is no less damaging than the New Right's similar view. This blame perpetuates a plague mentality, especially when one gay man becomes the principal target.

Patient Zero was how the CDC referred to him, and Randy Shilts made this moniker for Gaeten Dugas a household name with the publication of *And the Band Played On* in 1987; the 1993 HBO movie of Shilts' book kept his fame alive. A scientist at the CDC had been conducting a case history in the early 1980s in order to link people together with this new immune disorder in Los Angeles, San Francisco, and New York City. All of the AIDS cases seemed to intersect in their contact with the Canadian airline steward Dugas. Man after man the CDC talked with either had sexual contact with Dugas or with someone else who did. The main researcher on this case study was able to connect 40 men with AIDS in ten cities with Dugas, the supposed epicenter of this epidemiological occurrence.[33]

On the one hand, Shilts included the CDC's case study from the early 1980s in an effort to show the extant methods of scientific inquiry for discovering the cause of AIDS. Dugas, after all, "played a key role in spreading the new virus from one end of the United States to the other," Shilts concludes when he reports Dugas' death from AIDS in 1984.[34] But Dugas was not the only one who participated in sharing this new virus that Shilts, at times, leads us to believe. In addition, Shilts' chapter devoted to *Patient Zero* is in Part IV of his book entitled "The Gathering Darkness" with an epigraph from Camus' *The Plague*.[35] Discussing this patient as the CDC's focal point of transmission in a section of his book that ominously frames the imminent appearance of AIDS within the context of plague steers readers toward viewing Dugas as *the* primeval plague carrier. In reality, everyone Dugas had sex with was also involved in unwittingly transmitting the virus to other partners, or as Kinsella makes clear in his book on AIDS and the media when he critiques Shilts' presentation of Dugas, no single person was responsible for the spread of the disease.[36] Shilts does grant a small defense for Dugas when he reports Dugas' response to Dr. Conant's admonishment for him to have safer sex. After all, Dugas tells the doctor, "somebody gave this thing to me." But in the same breath, Shilts' defense is undercut by giving us Dugas' reminder to Dr. Conant that he will not "give up sex" and therefore will continue to spread the pestilence, as he sees it.[37]

Shilts' inclusion of Dugas' refusal to stop having sex while carrying this disease—along with further mentioning the circulating rumors on Castro Street in San Francisco that Dugas always announced, after having sex with someone in any given bath house, "I've got gay cancer. I'm going to die and so are you"—certainly stamps the placement of blame on this one gay man as the ultimate cause of the disease's spread.[38] Yet it is perhaps too harsh to view Shilts' portrayal of Dugas as the "personification of motiveless malignity," as one critic sees it.[39] "Motiveless malignity" was a phrase coined by the romantic poet Samuel Taylor Coleridge to describe the supposed evilness of Shakespeare's character Iago in *Othello*. If anything, these rumors about Dugas on Castro Street revealed one motive for Dugas' revelation of his disease to those he has sex with: jealousy of men who are not ill.

Although Shilts essentially ends up scapegoating one gay man as the human cause of AIDS, he actually spends more time presenting the bigger and ultimate cause: the U.S. government. AIDS "was allowed to happen by an array of institutions, all of which failed to perform their appropriate tasks to safeguard the public health," Shilts declares.[40] He sees the government's lack of funding to various institutions, including the CDC and NIH, for working toward the discovery of the organism that causes AIDS, the intercontinental scientific bickering over ownership of the eventual viral cause, and mostly Reagan's neglect in discussing the disease with our nation, all contributing to spreading AIDS across America.

Proposing human causes for an infectious disease positions AIDS as a plague and Shilts is not shy about using plague discourse throughout his book. In his "Prologue" alone, AIDS is described as "the tide of death," "pestilence," and "homosexual affliction."[41] The first section of the book opens with the quote from the book of the Apocalypse describing the pale horse, Death, which not only reminds us of Katherine Anne Porter's early twentieth-century short story detailing the 1918 influenza pandemic viewed as a plague by her, but obviously takes us back to the New Testament in which plague is presented as a divine corrective.[42] Shilts securely places AIDS within the global plague narrative.

Shilts primarily views AIDS as a plague that was caused by the government because 36,000 Americans contracted the disease and more than 20,000 died from it when Reagan finally publically addressed it for the first time in 1987.[43] Gay men, in particular, were victims of a deadly disease in Shilts' view because "the one nation with the knowledge, the resources, and the institutions to respond to the epidemic, had failed." Our country's "ignorance and fear, prejudice and rejection" of gay people provided the explanation for the government's neglect in addressing and funding the AIDS crisis in its early years.[44]

Larry Kramer also saw the government's inaction as one of the primary human causes of AIDS. "The Plague Years" captures one of his views of AIDS and it was published on the day of Reagan's first AIDS speech to the American people. Kramer was skeptical about any effectiveness the president's delayed response to the epidemic would have, and he supports his skepticism by revealing an interview with a Reagan administrator who admitted that

"Washington, D.C. is not interested in AIDS."[45] Kramer sees the government's lack of investment in AIDS as responsible for its high mortality rate and plague status.

Kramer essentially views Reagan's persistent unwillingness to actively fight the epidemic as "genocide" of AIDS victims.[46] This "genocide," a few weeks later, when Kramer speaks at a Gay Pride weekend crowd in Boston, becomes Reagan's "holocaust." The thousands upon thousands of men dying or dead could have been prevented if Reagan would have done something, anything, to help stop the disease's spread. "AIDS is our holocaust and Reagan is our Hitler. New York City is our Auschwitz," Kramer proclaims to this crowd.[47] These are strong accusations.

If the president had at least publically addressed AIDS earlier than 1987, public fear and a growing hysteria might have been quelled or at least diminished. Perhaps if Reagan had allocated more funds to the NIH and the CDC, viable treatments would have been found earlier than the 1990s. Perhaps if educational programs regarding prevention of HIV would have been developed earlier, fewer people would have contracted the disease. Because none of these actions occurred and the gay male community lost so many members, especially in urban areas, political activists like Kramer viewed this period as extermination, a plague that needlessly happened.

But Kramer also holds his own community responsible as one cause of AIDS' persistence. In his speech in Boston for Gay Pride weekend, he announces, "I'm tired of you, by your own passivity, actively participating in your own genocide."[48] He lambastes gay people for not giving enough money to organizations that support AIDS victims, for not raising enough money to procure an AIDS lobbyist on Capitol Hill, and for not volunteering at any gay organizations, to name a few peccadilloes. His message was intended to inspire his community to act, but for very different reasons Kramer perpetuates the more religiously and politically conservative notion that gay men were responsible for this disease, a view that many Americans shared. Kramer's blame might have inadvertently fed discrimination toward the gay community in people who already saw gay men as plague vectors.

To a substantial degree, anger became a more pervasive reaction to AIDS from within the gay community during this period, thanks to Kramer and other activists. Kramer spoke to a crowd in New York City in March 1987 highlighting the growth of AIDS cases to 32,000 from the 1,112 cases only four years before. He pleads with this crowd, "How long does it take before you get angry and fight back?"[49] He does not feel that the gay community is angry enough to unite and fight the FDA that Kramer holds responsible for the slow release of any promising new AIDS drugs. But Kramer remains inspired to act by his anger. Soon after this speech, ACT

UP—AIDS Coalition to Unleash Power—was formed by several activists, including Kramer, with the main goal of provoking governmental organizations to expedite the release of experimental drugs. Near the end of March 1987, ACT UP demonstrated against the FDA on Wall Street by hanging an effigy of the organization's head and distributing information about the snail-paced drug approval process.[50]

A less overtly angry response to AIDS came in the form of a slogan created for a poster by several gay activists who strategically plastered it on the face of buildings throughout New York City. **Silence = Death** appeared against a black background with a pink triangle arranged above the powerful phrase.[51] These activists took the inverted pink triangles that gay people were forced to wear in the concentration camps during World War II and placed the figure upright above the slogan. The cooptation of the Nazis' symbol for gays as marked for death signifies a new era for gay people. They refuse the same fate that would happen if certain institutions continued to refuse to recognize the severity of AIDS. I must admit that when I came across a **Silence = Death** pin in a downtown book shop in the fall of 1987, I fastened it to my purse and wore it proudly for years.

Yet other people reacted with silence to AIDS when it affected them personally or their loved ones because they feared the discrimination that was generated as a result of AIDS being perceived as a plague. The surgeon general understood this discrimination when he defended confidentiality for people with AIDS in his *Report*. He explained that people with the disease "are reluctant to be identified with AIDS because of the stigma that has been associated with it."[52] Paul Monette illustrates this stigma when Roger's brother, Sheldon, suggests hiding Roger's AIDS diagnosis from their parents initially but mostly from his law firm because "AIDS was as rife with terror and scapegoats as any launched by Rome."[53] Several of my patients lost their jobs when they were honest enough to reveal their diagnosis to supervisors or even when they started losing weight. This public denial of a disease occurred in 1665 when some Londoners attempted to avoid quarantining by lying about plague as the cause of death in relatives and in official reports denying plague as the cause of death in 1894 Hong Kong.

By the late 1980s, the plague-making of AIDS in American society also inspired a culture of death similar to the one in fourteenth-century Europe when bubonic plague killed more than half of the population. AIDS came nowhere near killing half of the American population during this time or since then, but again in urban communities, such as New York City and San Francisco, where AIDS was so prevalent, it felt like death was ubiquitous.

One reaction to this death was hedonism, as we saw in the Middle Ages. Although Shilts points out that several gay men in San Francisco responded to AIDS in a more ascetic vein by attending gay Alcoholics Anonymous meetings and dry clubs, others kept going to the parties "oblivious to the plague around them."[54] The survivors of this culturally constructed plague, like Boccaccio's, also attempted to forget about it through self-indulgent activities.

Despair seemed to usurp hedonism, though, as a more prevalent reaction to the death from AIDS. Carol Pogash captures some pretty dire perspectives when she reports on San Francisco General Hospital's treatment of AIDS throughout the 1980s. One patient who entered the emergency room there in 1989 announced that "everyone's going to die of AIDS anyway" when she abruptly pulled out her IV at the nurses' station, which resulted in a spray of her blood.[55] The Italian chronicler Agnolo di Tura expressed this despairing view after burying his own children who died from bubonic plague in the 1340s.

Although the newly emerging genre of AIDS "activist art" in the late 1980s could be classified as "agitprop" because it delivered a more blatantly political message than traditional art, its main subject was often despair over dying from this illness.[56] The photographer Nicholas Nixon, for example, captures the physical deterioration of a man with AIDS, Tom Moran, over a short period of time. In November 1987, Tom sits on his bed bare-chested and staring at the camera. His skeletal upper torso foregrounds the picture and not surprisingly his face expresses no emotion. In January 1988, Tom lies in his hospital bed even more emaciated; bearing the same expressionless face, only maybe there is a hint of sorrow. One month later, presumably in the same hospital bed, the close up of his face with its bony prominences outshining any other feature and his stained white lips—stained from the Mycelex troches patients popped in their mouths with some assistance up to five times daily in order to help combat oral yeast infections—conveys that any hope of escaping death has evaporated as Tom withers away to nothing.[57]

The famous, or as many people would say *infamous*, photographer Robert Mapplethorpe, who was notorious for his brisk photographs of naked people captured in compromising sadomasochistic positions, suffered from AIDS and released one last *Self-Portrait* in 1988 before his death. The artist's illness is evident in this photo as his gaunt face intently stares at the camera, revealing a deep fear of the unknown and perhaps a longing to stop suffering. His black garb and strategically chosen skull walking cane that he clutches reveal his forced march to the grave.[58] Like artists depicted plague many centuries before with the figure of Death dancing in their paintings, Mapplethorpe's last self-portrait is a still life of the personification of Death. Even Shilts personifies death in his book when he forecasts the appearance of AIDS on the morning of the Gay Pride parade in San Francisco in June 1980. "To be sure," he says, "Death was already elbowing its way through the crowds on that sunny morning."[59]

The death culture surrounding AIDS, like that surrounding bubonic plague, also entailed a fairly severe fear of contagion even in the late 1980s when we securely knew how the virus was transmitted. An article published near the end of 1987 revealed that Connecticut funeral homes were charging more money to prepare the bodies of AIDS victims and some simply did not accept the bodies at all. Sharon L. Bass interviewed some of these funeral directors who "expressed fear that the AIDS virus survives many hours after a person dies."[60] Even if the virus did survive that long, the precautions that funeral directors always used anyway with the dead infected with hepatitis would suffice. An extreme fear of contagion is evident in this group of professionals who now treat HIV as more contagious than hepatitis B, which it is not, and this fear drives their discriminatory treatment of the decedents.

Paul Monette describes his dental hygienist's reaction to him when he tells her honestly for her own protection that he was exposed to HIV: The hygienist "backed away in abject horror and ran from the room."[61] Today's omnipresent practice of dental staff donning gloves and masks for all patients, regardless of their HIV status, was not common in the late 1980s. Like this health-care professional, the chief orthopedic surgeon at San Francisco General Hospital exhibited an extreme fear of contagion of AIDS patients. According to Pogash, this surgeon wanted all of her patients to be tested for HIV before she operated on them, and she thought that HIV possibly could be transmitted through sweat, which it cannot be. She mentioned this route of viral transmission to a group of already scared public pool directors and parents of handicapped children who did not want AIDS patients swimming in their pool.[62]

Furthermore, in 1989 this surgeon appeared on national TV to perform surgery with the astronaut-like garb of personal protection that she created in order to avoid contracting HIV during any operation. She actually told *60 Minutes* that operating on patients with HIV posed the same risk as having anal intercourse.[63] Some of the surgeon's colleagues discerned that "the real issue" behind her actions and statements "was her fear of the disease."[64] It was one thing for an extreme fear of contagion to affect the general public, but when it gripped the medical community that cared for AIDS patients and potential HIV carriers, we are at the heart of witnessing the irrationality produced when a disease is perceived as plague. This community was the one that was supposed to be rational and objective in delivering medical care to anyone who needed it.

This fear of contagion within the medical community continued to be accompanied by projected disdain. Even Robert Gallo in his January 1987 article on the AIDS virus admits that "in the past two decades one of the fondest boasts of medical science has been the conquest of infectious diseases," in well-developed countries at least.[65] Gallo recognizes that this view was pure pride that was struck down by the growing presence of HIV. Those in the medical field who held this conquering view of microbes may have projected their disdain of defeat onto AIDS patients they encountered and treated.

The mainstream press covered the lay perspective of medicine's failure to conquer infectious diseases. The 1987 *Newsweek* article that referred to the AIDS epidemic as a plague year mentions that the pervasive spirit of optimism that is characteristic of Americans in general renders them "unaccustomed to an epidemic that resists the magic of our medicine."[66] Americans having to face that AIDS broke the spell of our medical advances in the late twentieth century may have felt a disdain of this failure that was projected onto AIDS victims.

Fear and disdain of this disease continued to contribute to varying degrees of scapegoating. For example, when Reagan finally conceded to the need for a commission to address AIDS public policy in early May 1987, the issues discussed by the White House overlooked prevention efforts and instead focused on outing those people who carried HIV. The president's spokesperson made it clear that this executively sanctioned AIDS panel would "recommend ways to protect Americans who do not have the disease." But these "ways" did not include safer sex or needle exchange programs. One policy considered was mandatory testing in order "to determine who is carrying the AIDS virus," and confidentiality was absent from the discussion.[67] From the White House's perspective, the public revelation of the HIV positive person simply would be justified in their efforts to protect *disease-free* Americans.

When we really consider, from a scientific and not a plague-imbibed point of view, how HIV is *only* transmitted via the exchange of infected bodily fluids and not through the air, how exactly would mandatory testing benefit the uninfected? If I know someone is HIV positive, I can avoid having sexual intercourse or sharing a needle with that person. Suppose that person tested HIV negative but had not developed antibodies to the virus at the moment of testing and now is positive at the moment of fluid exchange? Safe sex and using a clean needle for injecting drugs would have done far more toward solving the problem of protecting supposedly disease-free Americans, like it does now.

If mandatory testing would have become a reality in the 1980s, the HIV positive would have been brandished with a scarlet letter. After all, men only perceived to be gay and Haitian people in America during this decade were already marked by virtue of their status as risk groups for AIDS regardless of their individual HIV status. They suffered acts of hatred and discrimination *because* they were viewed as potential plague carriers.

Although mandatory testing for HIV never came to fruition, the proposal for it with the government's objective of protecting Americans from HIV scapegoats those who do carry the virus. The HIV positive carry the onus for the spread of the disease, instead of everyone carrying it when engaging in any behavior that could result in viral transmission. Susan Sontag warned that knowledge of anyone's HIV positive status creates a "new class of lifetime pariahs: the future ill."[68] This is the reason why activists in many communities have always fought for confidential testing. HIV positive people did not want to be viewed by employers as sitting in Death's waiting room, or worse, risking the possibility of being placed on a "list" only to enter some sort of camp for the ill. This risk was Monette's justification for not even getting tested for HIV when he discovered his low T4 cell lymphocyte count, the harbinger of his illness.[69]

An even more overt form of scapegoating than the proposed mandatory HIV testing at this time was Jesse Helms's successful legal efforts to prevent federal funding for education about AIDS that had anything to do with gay sexual activities, and especially his enacted ban on travel to the United States for HIV positive persons. Helms, a U.S. senator for several decades until his death in 2008, attached his infamous amendment to a large spending bill going through Congress near the end of 1987. His religious and political alignment with the New Right certainly influenced his proposals. He was appalled by a GMHC pamphlet he read that included safe sex education for gay men. He immediately introduced legislation that prevented any federal funding for this type of education while pontificating to the Senate, "every Christian ethic cries out for me to do something."[70] Helms' legalized discrimination of denying funding that would help gay men stem this deadly illness at this time seems to defy at least one Christian ethic: love your neighbor as you would yourself. But Helms' motivations were not derived from a place of love; they came from a place of disdain for gays, a disdain that perhaps was projected onto them because of the self-hatred he might have experienced over needing to be saved (one of the central beliefs of born-again Christians).

The ban on travel of HIV positive persons to the United States that found its way into the Helms' amendment certainly was influenced by the country's fear of contagion in 1987. This ban, in essence, scapegoated the HIV positive abroad for the potential spread of AIDS here. By admitting one's HIV positive status on a visa application or waiver form, entrance to this country was denied. This law was international quarantining. In July 2009, one such potential HIV positive traveler from England was denied entrance to the United States for a speaking engagement at a health-care conference on the West Coast. He reports that the actual question about HIV status on the visa waiver form "was alongside those asking if he was a terrorist or a Nazi."[71] It seems that our country had categorized people with HIV/AIDS as weapons of mass destruction. President George W. Bush began the process of lifting this travel ban in 2008, and President Barack Obama finished the job in early 2010 when the ban was finally obliterated.[72]

Domestic quarantining of HIV positive persons was proposed in the late 1980s but never was sanctioned legally. These proposals also stem more from a place of discrimination than of public health concern. Quarantining AIDS patients would not have resulted in public safety like the 1665 London one did to a degree. Unlike bubonic disease, HIV is not transmitted via air droplets or by touching flea-infested garments. California entertained quarantine on one of its ballots at this time.[73] No doubt cases like the one in Fresno, in which a known HIV positive woman admitted to her counselor that she still engaged in unsafe sex as a prostitute and shared needles when using drugs, fueled the proposal. The counselor at least questioned whether or not quarantining even would be beneficial considering AIDS does not go away like the flu.[74] Should HIV positive people then be quarantined for their life span?

Helms and Pat Robertson, the televangelist who ran for president during this time, not surprisingly favored quarantining AIDS patients. One journalist who covered the quarantine issue said America needs to decide whether to treat AIDS "as a disease, calling forth compassion and support, or a moral issue, a *plague* whose victims are pariahs."[75] Proposals for quarantining AIDS patients arise from the view that the disease is a plague spread by casual contact, especially by the marginalized groups of people who have been held responsible for it. In reality, AIDS is not spread by casual contact and everyone is responsible for preventing its transmission.

Scapegoating in the form of displays of hatred for victims of diseases created as plagues remained a reality in the late 1980s. The burning of Jews who were blamed for bubonic plague in fourteenth-century Germany was a misdirected punishment that did not only belong to that dark past. In Arcadia, Florida, when three young HIV positive hemophiliac boys were allowed to return to school after being banned for their illness, their parents, the Rays, endured death threats and other parents boycotting the Ray boys' presence by keeping their own children home from school. The Rays' home was burnt to the ground at the conclusion of their sons' first week back at school. Thankfully, only the children's uncle was at the Rays' home at the time of the fire, and he escaped. The boys' father saw fear of AIDS generating this act of hatred. He told reporters that "educational leaders and politicians had let panic rule the community and had failed to educate the public," especially in regard to HIV not being transmitted casually.[76]

A lack of education in places of employment regarding how HIV is transmitted also contributed to more subtle displays of hatred such as shunning people known to have the disease. In early 1989, this evasive behavior abounded in the community of Long Island, New York. The director of an educational program for AIDS there revealed that "most businesses still deny that AIDS is a problem on the Island," and therefore there is a paucity of educational programs in the workplace. One high school teacher with AIDS, for example, did not feel comfortable enough to reveal his diagnosis to his fellow teachers when he ended up on disability. As a matter of fact, when he did not correct their assumptions that he had cancer, he received support and sympathy from them.[77]

An employee at a medical laboratory in Long Island actually expressed that he experienced "the silent plague" when his fellow employees learned about his AIDS diagnosis.[78] His colleagues would not mention the word *AIDS* and they told their manager they did not want to work with this man. Subsequently, this employee with AIDS was placed on a different shift. One can only imagine how warm his welcome was on the new shift. Granted this man was not terminated from his job when his disease was made public—a frequent occurrence during this period even when AIDS was only suspected—but the willful isolation he experienced from his community of workers *because* of his illness demonstrates the perpetual power of plague-making.

CHAPTER 8

Living with Plague (1990–1994)

She was a late admission, sometime after 11 P.M. "Gina, did you hear Freddie had it, too? He died today," Stephanie's husband frantically announced to me in the hallway of our unit as the transporter wheeled her stretcher with such zeal like he was attempting to escape a haunted house. I initially cared for Stephanie in mid-1991 when she was first diagnosed with AIDS and cryptococcal meningitis—an unpleasant fungal infection of the brain that preys on people with weakened immune systems. None of us could ever remain too frustrated with Stephanie then for being a little particular about the way she took her dozen medications a few times a day—one pill at a time with exactly three sips of water, only through the big blue straw she brought with her from home. After all, she had to endure the dreaded daily treatment for her meningitis: intravenous Amphotericin B, or "shake and bake," as nurses nicknamed it for its pronounced, and almost guaranteed, side-effects of chills and high fevers.

Now Stephanie was being admitted again with a recurrence of the infection. Al, her husband, was quite upset with the neglectful treatment she received in the emergency room (ER) that he attributed to her diagnosis. Stephanie was there almost 48 hours—not an unusual wait in a New York City ER at this time—but she was not offered a meal tray during that time or any pain medications for the intense headache produced by the brain infection. She also lay in her own urine because no one offered her a bedpan. Al saw a correlation between their experience and Freddie Mercury's, the talented singer and songwriter for the rock group Queen, as he could not stop talking about how the British press treated him. The press attempted to force Mercury's AIDS diagnosis into the public arena in spite of the singer's consistent denials.[1] Anyone who was a fan of the group watched Freddie's facial bones grow more and more pronounced as he lost pound after pound with each stage performance. Most of his fans kind of figured he had AIDS but really just lamented another great artist stolen by the disease instead of looking for public confirmation of it.

It is unbelievable, yet understandable, that Freddie Mercury did not release the news of his illness until the day before he died on November 24, 1991. AIDS had been around for a decade and still this rock star did not feel comfortable enough to discuss his disease publically, no doubt for fear of discrimination. A decade into the epidemic, many medical staff members treating patients, like Stephanie, still barely entered their rooms and subjected them to the same treatment as a prisoner of war would have experienced, or, in this case, a perceived plague victim.[2]

In 1989 alone, some 23,000 people had died from AIDS in the United States and 90 percent of those diagnosed before 1984 had died.[3] The number of AIDS cases in women had increased "from 9 percent in early 1987 to 11 percent in 1989," which explained why I started to care for more and more women like Stephanie.[4] Yet these statistics for women are slightly deceptive, especially when we consider, as Gina Corea did in *The Invisible Epidemic*, how women were neglected by the CDC and other medical institutions when it came to diagnosing AIDS. Corea points out that "gynecological symptoms of the disease were found in women but were never added to the AIDS surveillance definition."[5] The definition she refers to was originally developed by the CDC and revised in 1987.[6] It detailed what diseases indicated an AIDS diagnosis, and gynecological ones were not a part of the definition. Severe vaginal yeast infections, for example, and cervical cancer were not even considered relevant to a woman's HIV status. Most doctors did not even test women for HIV antibodies with these conditions. These conditions, as Corea argues, were not experienced by men with HIV/AIDS and therefore were neglected as possible AIDS-defining illnesses. The statistics for women with AIDS at this time were grossly underestimated.

Corea's book, however, was published in 1992, one year before the CDC released its updated AIDS surveillance definition, a definition still used today. The 1993 definition included vaginal yeast infections, cervical dysplasia (abnormal cell growth in the cervix), cervical cancer, and even pelvic inflammatory disease as indicative of AIDS in the presence of HIV antibodies.[7] The inclusion of these diseases increased the female AIDS caseload even more.

African Americans were also becoming a more prominent presence in the overall number of AIDS cases in America. According to Phillip Brian Harper, from June 1981 until February 1991 there were 167,803 people with AIDS and 38,361 of them were African American males.[8] In New York City alone, "blacks comprised nearly a third of the 36,000 AIDS cases" reported through the end of 1991. And the *MMWR* confirmed a 5 percent increase in AIDS cases among blacks from 1987 to 1989.[9]

Women and blacks had AIDS from the beginning of the epidemic along-side gay white males, but now with their numbers measurably increasing in the early 1990s the gay white male was finally being dethroned as the quintessential AIDS sufferer. In the media, people other than Rock Hudson and Liberace were a focus. Elizabeth Glaser, the *Starsky and Hutch* star's wife, and Mary Fisher, a wealthy Republican, spoke publically about their AIDS diagnosis. The basketball player Magic Johnson announced his HIV positive status in November 1991. He stressed that some woman from his past must have given him the virus.[10] I especially remember his announcement because our unit was inundated with calls that night from men revealing unpro-tected sexual encounters with women and asking us for reassurance about their chances of getting AIDS. Arthur Ashe, the black tennis professional, openly struggled with AIDS and died from it in early 1993.

It took a decade into the epidemic for women to unite and speak out about how AIDS was affecting them. Many women with AIDS by the early 1990s were taking political action in order to be included as participants in the new clinical trials for antiretroviral medications to halt the replication of HIV.[11] Most women had been excluded from research based on the fact that they had child-bearing potential. Study doctors were afraid to pose any risk to a potential fetus by allowing women to take these drugs. Near the end of 1991, some women actually chained themselves to a building at the CDC and demanded a change in the definition of AIDS so that it would include the gynecological diseases so many of them had been experiencing since they became HIV positive.[12]

African Americans, like women with AIDS, responded more slowly than gay men in addressing AIDS within their communities. By mid-1989 in New York City with blacks comprising 33 percent of the AIDS cases, black clergymen finally began to preach about the impact of AIDS. "Churches and mosques are considered the most influential institutions in black neigh-borhoods," one journalist points out, and therefore can be used as a gauge for issues that are addressed in the community.[13] And by 1992 with close to 50 percent of minority urban populations infected with AIDS and with Magic Johnson's public announcement of his HIV status, secular black leaders and lawmakers also began to address AIDS by seeking funding for programs.[14]

The long-standing marginalized status of women and blacks in American society certainly existed before the emergence of AIDS in our supposedly post-civil rights era. This marginalization may in part explain these commu-nities' slower response to AIDS. In addition, the U.S. medical community viewed gays, women, and blacks as "others," as Gina Corea insightfully notes, a perception that did not assist in empowering women and blacks to address

AIDS in their own communities.[15] The perception of "otherness" by people in positions of power—in this case, the power to treat the sick—facilitates blame of the victim of the disease, and the psychology of victimhood can impede action in the victims. Gay men were still marginalized but gay political advocacy groups that formed after Stonewall, coupled with the initial severe impact of AIDS on the urban gay male community, provoked an earlier united and forceful gay response to AIDS.

In the black community, it was difficult to admit the growing problem of AIDS because its members feared being "blamed for the disease, which is thought to have originated in Africa," as one journalist observes.[16] Haitians were viewed as a risk group based on nothing substantive except their ethnicity—of course, this ethnic profiling was never officially admitted—which helps to explain African Americans' fear of blame for the disease.

Furthermore, black communities in general, according to Phillip Brian Harper, did not feel comfortable discussing sexuality, let alone male homosexuality, subjects that are difficult to avoid when addressing AIDS. Harper mentions the old joke among blacks regarding AIDS: "There's good news and bad news. The bad news is I have AIDS, the good news is I'm an IV drug user."[17] AIDS carried the connotation of being a gay disease even a decade into the epidemic because of its initial presentation and reinforcement by the media and medical community as the gay plague. Even when the "gay" was dropped from the plague label in public discourse, people still perceived it as a primarily gay disease, as this joke suggests. But the general plague label for AIDS was not dropped by the early 1990s, which also explains why blacks and women were reluctant to discuss the impact of AIDS on their respective communities. No one wanted to be thought of as responsible for incurring this disease.

Mary Fisher, the HIV positive Republican, addressed the Republican National Convention in August 1992 and admonished fellow partisans "who have regarded AIDS as a self-inflicted plague earned by immoral behavior."[18] Fisher experienced this judgment for the disease firsthand, even though she was not a gay male or IVDU. She explained to Frank Rich during an interview a few years later that there was "a continuing stigmatization of people with AIDS, especially gay men." Although Rich's article revealed his admiration for this woman living with HIV, it was couched in the very plague discourse that produced the stigmatization experienced by Fisher and others living with the disease. Rich said he was amazed "by yet another life that has blossomed in the plague."[19]

In *Plague Doctors: Responding to the AIDS Epidemic in France and America*, anthropologist and physician Jamie L. Feldman discusses how naming diseases guides how we view them within and outside the medical field.

She says that "naming is perhaps the first and most common step in making meaning of any experience."[20] Her logic helps us understand that when GRID was the name for AIDS it meant that it was a gay disease. Feldman, however, does not address the implication of the "naming of AIDS" as a plague by writers and fellow physicians. Furthermore, she endorses the importance of metaphors in medicine for the purpose of "making sense of experience."[21] Feldman's metaphorical usage of "plague" to "name" the very doctors caring for AIDS patients throughout her book, without analyzing the detrimental implications of this label, inadvertently perpetuates the fear of the disease and blame for its victims that has accompanied the word *plague* for centuries.

In 1990 Larry Kramer still felt like "we are living in a time of plague" because hundreds of cases continued to be diagnosed daily, hundreds of people with AIDS died daily, and two presidents did not work hard enough to stop the disease's spread through massive funding and education.[22] Even five years later when journalist Felicia R. Lee showcased a nurse at The Robert Mapplethorpe Residential Treatment Facility in lower Manhattan—a long-term care home for AIDS patients funded with money from the photographer's estate—she described the nurse's daily commute from New Jersey to New York City as "travel into the heart of the great plague of the twentieth century."[23] New York in 1995 carried 70,000 AIDS cases, with the average AIDS patient presented now as an economically and socially disadvantaged drug user.[24] For Kramer and Lee, inside an urban center, AIDS is a plague and even *the* plague based on the geographically concentrated high number of people infected.

Similarly, out on the Fire Island Pines, a beach-vacationing community on Long Island a few hours from the city, the typically 80 percent summer gay population dwindled considerably by 1993. Diane Ketchum describes AIDS as being "like the bubonic plague" in this popular summer destination spot. AIDS warrants the comparison for this journalist because there are deaths reported weekly among the returning summer denizens.[25]

Ketcham's simile for AIDS (bubonic plague) carries on the lineage between the highly infectious, fatal plague of yore and AIDS, a lineage also perpetuated within the Catholic Church and the arts during this time. When Peter Steinfels covered the paucity of applicants entering the Catholic religious orders in the early 1990s and the confused sense of their mission within the church, he comments on one group of clerics who still have a clear purpose. The Alexian brothers are "an order founded in the Middle Ages to care for plague victims who are now helping people with AIDS."[26] These priests obviously view AIDS as a modern bubonic plague and they remain committed to their heritage of caring for its victims.

The medieval past of plague does not escape the stage either when AIDS is the subject. *Angels in America* by Tony Kushner was performed in two parts in the first half of the 1990s. One of the main characters, Prior, who suffers from AIDS is visited by dead relatives who suffered from diseases called plagues in past centuries. His thirteenth-century British squire relative (Prior 1) notices that Prior takes pills "for the pestilence," but stresses that bubonic plague was worse in his time. Yet bubonic plague and AIDS are conflated in this family lineage of suffered diseases when Prior 1 pronounces, "in a family as long-descended as the Walters, there are bound to be a few carried off by plague."[27]

Writings and films in the early-to-mid-1990s continued to capture and circulate the view that AIDS had divine and human causes as opposed to solely focusing on the well-known viral one. Douglas Crimp and Adam Rolston critique the Catholic Church's view and treatment of AIDS in their 1990 piece, "Stop the Church." New York City's archbishop, Cardinal O'Conner, would not concede to a national bishop conference's suggestion to lift the ban on condom usage in an effort to halt the spread of HIV. O'Conner, like Reagan, inadvertently contributed to the proliferation of HIV infection by upholding dogma that precluded safe sexual practices.

In addition, disallowing the practice of safe sex with condoms indicates that those clerics who did so were not secure in believing that HIV transmission was the cause of AIDS; rather sexual behaviors that ultimately incurred divine punishment were the cause. One theologian attending the Vatican's first conference on AIDS actually endorsed this view when he "suggested that AIDS could indeed be seen as God's wrath against homosexuality."[28] Within this perspective, safe sex cannot hinder viral transmission but a blockade on homosexuality can because that would appease God.

Cruelty toward AIDS patients was also justified by those who viewed the disease as divine punishment for a certain sexual orientation. O'Conner's insistence on banning condoms influenced the media's reticence about advertising safe sexual practices, and this lack of advertising contributed to the growing number of AIDS cases. Open discussions about sexual practices were not commonplace at this time. Sex was still a taboo subject. Without the media's message of promotion of safer sex, many people clung to old unsafe and untold habits that ultimately facilitated the transmission of the virus. Leaders, like the bishop, could not see the cruelty in their lack of support for condom usage because they felt justified in their view that AIDS was a divine punishment for being gay. Condom ads were finally allowed on television in early 1994, and when they ran conservative factions, like the National Conference on Catholic Bishops, condemned them.[29]

Several black, conservative religious leaders blamed certain members of their own communities for AIDS. In 1991, one bishop commented that many of his conservative clergy colleagues "preach that AIDS" is "the plague upon the land because of disobedience."[30] This "disobedience" included what these church leaders perceived as sins, primarily homosexuality, sex outside of marriage, and drug use. Here in 1991, the culture of the Middle Ages lives on. People's "sins" were still being viewed as the cause of AIDS, just as they were viewed as responsible for bubonic plague.

One of the primary ramifications of blaming human actions for any disease, specifically those labeled as plagues, is silence on the part of people suffering from them. A pastor of one Baptist church in 1991 mentioned that one of her church members who had attended church her whole life and now has AIDS revealed her cancer diagnosis to others but not the other one because "she's afraid of what they'll think."[31] We have heard that refrain several times from the mouths of those living and dying with AIDS. Human behaviors may often be blamed for certain cancers, like cigarette smoking causing lung cancer, but cancer sufferers usually admit their diagnoses. But then again cancer has not been constructed as a plague as AIDS has been.

Some members of the gay community also continued to view their own sexual behaviors as the cause of AIDS. "The first mainstream American film" regarding AIDS released in 1990, *Longtime Companion*, at moments expresses this view. Although Vincent Canby described the movie as "insipid"—it is in many ways, especially in the superficial character development—and criticized its sole focus on the impact of AIDS on the gay white male community when by this time so many other communities were feeling the toll of AIDS, this movie, like other art forms, responds to and expresses the culture in which it was produced.[32] The viewer is granted access into the lives of several gay male couples who slowly have to deal with this new illness personally when the movie begins with the first reported cases of AIDS in the summer of 1981. The setting alternates between New York City and Fire Island, where by 1983 sallow faces and thin bodies painted with purple lesions replaced the buffed, tan ones that were once a part of the landscape of the beaches and walkways there.

One of the male characters articulates the too familiar self-blaming view of AIDS, as the 1990s open. Friends gathered on the deck of a beach house observe an ill-looking man stroll by and this character criticizes fellow gay men who have too much sex and use too many drugs. The sole female character he vents to defends these men by reminding him that "it is a virus" that causes AIDS and not this behavior. "I know it's a virus and so is the black plague, but not everybody got that," he retorts.[33] Of course, we know that bubonic disease is caused by a bacterium and not a virus, but the cultural myths surrounding plague in general persist here. Most significant, his statement implies that people in the medieval era, as in our own so-called plague time, could control whether or not they were struck with the illness by modifying their "sinful" behaviors.

Viewing certain behaviors as the cause of AIDS is also reinforced within the context of plague in Kushner's *Angels in America*. When Prior, Kushner's main character with AIDS, receives his visit from relatives who have died from different diseases referred to as plagues, their conversation reveals that the twentieth-century Prior with AIDS is gay. They go on to discuss how each of them contracted their own brand of plague. Prior 2 acknowledges that his illness came "from a water pump"—a reference to the cholera epidemic in nineteenth-century London—and Prior 1's medieval plague "came from fleas"—a reference to bubonic disease. Prior 2 then attributes Prior's AIDS to his homosexuality. He declares, "I understand [your plague] is the lamentable consequence of venery."[34] This verbal exchange between past victims of diseases considered plagues and the current living victim of a disease considered a plague not only embodies the American view of the first decade of the AIDS epidemic that certain people, namely gays, were punished for their behavior with this disease, but reinforces the place of AIDS in the global plague narrative.

When *Philadelphia* was released in 1993 to a wider viewing audience than *Longtime Companion*, it actually reflected and presented more tolerant views of AIDS. Yet alongside these views were persistent discriminatory ones that placed blame on the disease's victims. The eponymous title of the movie suggests that if anyone with AIDS will be treated with fairness, it will happen in the City of Brotherly Love. After all, this is where the Declaration of Independence and Constitution, documents that theoretically ensure each American's right to equality, were endorsed. And the movie does depict Andy Beckett receiving this equal treatment in spite of his AIDS and KS diagnoses, which were still stigmatizing ones at this time. Not only does Andy's Philadelphian family express genuine concern about his doctor appointments and T cell counts, they embrace him and his partner. At a family event celebrating his parents' fortieth wedding anniversary, family members hug and kiss Andy freely and Andy holds a baby just like everyone else. The sister in *An Early Frost* would not allow Michael to even be near her children or her unborn baby.

But this nondiscriminating and rational treatment of the AIDS victim does not follow Andy outside of this cozy, private space. In the early 1990s, most employees with AIDS anywhere still did not feel comfortable freely revealing their diagnosis and neither does Andy. His law firm, however, suspects his diagnosis because of his thinning frame and visible KS lesion. In spite of making him a senior associate before his AIDS is suspected, the law firm terminates him based on specious allegations of an "attitude problem" and "grogginess" at the office. At the court trial, the major focus of the movie where Andy attempts to sue his firm for prejudicial treatment, the prevalent American view that gay men cause AIDS comes to the forefront in the law firm's accusations. The lead lawyer for the firm reminds Andy that he was "duplicitous" in concealing his disease—an irony indeed because he probably would have been fired anyway if he admitted he had AIDS. This firm lawyer then blames Andy's "lifestyle and reckless behavior" as the cause of his disease.[35]

The old guilty – innocent distinction between AIDS victims is reinforced in the movie when Andy's law firm asks one of its female employees with AIDS to testify on their behalf. Her continual employment with the firm, in spite of her diagnosis, purportedly supports their position of nondiscriminating treatment of people with AIDS. This woman was not fired but she contracted AIDS through a blood transfusion before the blood supply was tested for HIV antibodies in the early 1980s. The law firm's defense highlights how her behavior did not cause AIDS. And another witness called forth by the firm solidifies the distinction between those with AIDS who should be blamed, like Andy, and those who contract it "innocently," like this woman.[36]

Unlike the so-called "innocent" female at Andy's court trial, many women with AIDS at this time were blamed as the primary transmitters of HIV to their babies and not viewed as victims themselves. This view existed in spite of there being only a 30 percent chance of transmitting HIV to an unborn fetus, a somewhat encouraging statistic considering that the panoply of antiretroviral drugs that will decrease this chance even more was not available yet.[37]

Mothers with HIV being blamed as the cause of AIDS in their children is illustrated in Corea's portrait of a family struggling with the disease. One grandmother, Ada, has to deal with raising her three HIV positive grandchildren because her daughter is so ill from AIDS. Before Ada agrees to take on this enormous responsibility, she implies that her daughter was responsible for her grandchildren's disease even though her daughter did not know her husband had AIDS. Ada thinks, "I didn't bring this on! I didn't make these children sick! So why should I get involved?"[38] Ada's daughter did not make these children sick either; rather the virus did without her permission.

One of the more dangerous views of AIDS causality that emerged in the early 1990s questioned and even denied HIV as the cause and instead proposed certain behaviors. Robert Root-Bernstein, a Michigan State University physiology professor, proposed in 1993, almost a decade after the viral discovery of AIDS, that HIV might not be the cause of AIDS. He arrived at this theory after teaching Koch's postulates in a biology course. He decided that because HIV "could not be isolated in pure form" and did not produce AIDS in lab monkeys infected with the virus, HIV may not be the cause of this disease.[39] Root-Bernstein was perhaps premature in noting that HIV could not be isolated in pure form because only a few short years later we were able to measure the number of HIV-RNA copies, or the actual viral particles, instead of just the antibodies to HIV. As for lab monkeys not developing AIDS in spite of being HIV positive, there are plenty of humans who have turned out to share this state as well. For not completely understood reasons, some primates remain HIV positive without developing full-blown AIDS, but this does not mean that HIV is not the cause of AIDS in those who do develop the disease.

In addition, Root-Bernstein views the CDC's statistics of "97.6 percent of all AIDS cases still falling within the risk groups established at the beginning of the plague" as proof that there is something other than a viral cause of AIDS.[40] If AIDS were truly caused by a virus, so this logic goes, it would not be contained within certain groups and would infect anyone. However, if we examine HIV infection from the standpoint that everyone living in America is a member of the general population and "risk groups" are an irrelevant construct because HIV is transmitted through "risky behavior," this scientist's argument collapses. A gay male is not at risk for HIV/AIDS *because* he is gay. He is at risk only when he engages in an unprotected sexual act that can potentially transmit the virus. An IV drug user is not at risk for HIV/AIDS *because* he shoots drugs. The drug abuser is at risk only when he shares needles with other users. The hemophiliac is not at risk for AIDS *because* he is Factor VIII deficient. He is only at risk if the clotting factor derived from blood donors is not HIV negative. The establishment of Haitians as a risk group by the CDC cuts to the heart of the problem with offering risk groups instead of risky behavior when it comes to HIV transmission. Being born Haitian is not a risk factor for contracting HIV/AIDS, even though epidemiologists at first intimated that it was. Haitians with the disease did not admit unsafe sexual or drug use practices. Their behavior and *not* who they are ethnically made some of them at risk for the disease.

Root-Bernstein ultimately believes there are other immunosuppressive factors besides infection with HIV, such as coinfection with other viruses, which could result in the disease state of AIDS. Fair enough. At least he acknowledges HIV in the mix. But what really ranks highest on his causality list is "an individual's behavior," but not just any *individual's* behavior.

Root-Bernstein proclaims that "healthy people do not get AIDS."[41] Yet, I have taken care of plenty of people who felt well and were not ill with any disease and contracted HIV and eventually developed AIDS. According to him, drug abuse and semen entering the blood stream through anal intercourse are the primary culprits for producing this weakened immune system that leads to AIDS. This professor seems to overlook other people with weakened immune systems, such as night shift workers whose altered circadian rhythms can produce lowered immunity and cancer patients undergoing chemotherapy, who do not develop AIDS. Furthermore, not everyone who uses drugs or engages in unprotected anal intercourse develops AIDS. HIV needs to be exchanged in order for this development to occur.

This prejudicial behavioral theory of AIDS causality, supported a few years later by another scientist, Peter Duesberg, is dangerous because it downplays and practically denies the viral cause of AIDS. This denial could influence straight, gay, or bisexual people to stop practicing any type of safe sex and could stop drug users from using clean needles. This denial could even theoretically lead to a moratorium on checking blood products for HIV antibodies. Why bother if HIV is not the cause of AIDS? Most notably, this type of behavioral theory facilitates the blame of already stigmatized groups, in particular gay men and IVDUs, for the existence and spread of AIDS.

This so-called scientific, or at least academic, type of doubt and denial about HIV causing AIDS fed even more denial in our culture at this time, most notably captured in the 1994 movie *KIDS*.[42] The unsympathetic, main character, Telly, sees his main goal in life as deflowering as many young girls as he can find. What he does not know is that he is carrying HIV, which he inadvertently passes to Jenny, another teenager who is astonished that he has HIV when she and her girlfriend responsibly get tested after having unprotected sex. Jenny has only had one sexual partner in her life—the wrong one. This is actually the movie's powerful message: It only takes one unprotected sexual encounter to contract HIV.

The movie's main focus is on the teenage boys' world of unprotected sex, promiscuity, getting high, and an unbelievable denial of AIDS, which has resulted in Jenny's HIV positive status. As Telly discusses his sexual conquests, especially of virgins whom he likes to make bleed, he bellows out that "condoms suck."[43] Another boy goes a step further and discredits the very existence of AIDS because he does not know anyone who died from the disease. He declares that AIDS "is made up."[44] The movie does not endorse this denial because its major narrative thread focuses on Jenny trying to find Telly in order to tell him that he gave her HIV before he has intercourse with another girl. Unfortunately, not only is Jenny too late as she finds Telly having intercourse at the most popular party of the night, but Telly's best friend, Casper, essentially rapes Jenny when she is passed out after the party's spirit has been depleted.

We feel afraid for these male kids, in particular, who are unwittingly transmitting HIV as a result of their denial about the disease's existence. The majority of their denial perhaps stems from a budding adolescent desire for unfettered sexual activity and experimentation, yet circulating theories, like Root-Bernstein's, could have contributed to this type of reckless behavior in our society, which the director, Larry Clark, depicts artistically. These kids, after all, are "healthy"—Root-Bernstein's protection against AIDS—because they do not engage in anal intercourse or use intravenous drugs. So why not have unprotected penile-vaginal sex?

Other cultural depictions of denial as a reaction to AIDS during this time stemmed from the disease's stigma as a gay disease. Roy Cohn in *Angels in America* was based on the real-life, powerful lawyer who not only worked for Senator McCarthy but instrumentally succeeded in obtaining the death penalty for Ethel and Julius Rosenberg, two known American communists who were falsely accused of espionage in the early 1950s. Cohn's denial of AIDS and his own death from it are major scenes in *Kushner's* play. When Roy's doctor initially gives him the diagnosis, he cannot accept it because, as he sees it, AIDS "afflicts mostly homosexuals and drug addicts."[45] And as Roy also sees it, he is not a drug addict or a homosexual, even though his doctor reminds him that he has treated Roy for several venereal diseases of the rectum in the past.

The discrimination against homosexuals in American society did not facilitate their political power. Perhaps the fact that gay marriage has only been deemed legal by our government in less than 10 states is the greatest testimony of this. Roy Cohn cannot admit that he has a disease that many of the powerless get. He comments that homosexuals in New York City cannot even get a simple antidiscrimination bill passed through the city government, whereas he can get the president of the United States on the phone anytime he wants. Therefore, Roy emphatically tells his doctor, "AIDS is what homosexuals have. I have liver cancer."[46] If AIDS had not been created as a plague in the 1980s, Roy Cohn's denial might not have been so tenacious. If attention to AIDS in the media and in medical writings in the 1980s would have focused equally on women, babies, blood product recipients, IVDUs, and all races, it might have been more difficult to facilely see the disease as a gay one.

Other reactions to AIDS as a plague in the first half of the 1990s can be understood as part of the death culture that continued to surround the disease. Anger over deaths in the gay community did not abate, especially anger toward the American government for its neglect in addressing the disease's spread. Larry Kramer pleas with his audience in his Introduction to *The Destiny of Me* to "not vote for any candidate who would allow AIDS to become a plague."[47] Ned Weeks's character throughout this drama is the voice of anger against the slow progress of the medical establishment in finding effective treatments for AIDS.

But the angriest reactions to the treatment of AIDS victims as plague carriers are found in the short film by Rosa von Praunheim, *Silence=Death*.[48] Dominated by the poet David Wojnarowicz's staccato, enraged readings about the discrimination experienced by people with AIDS, and interviews with other artists suffering from or affected by AIDS, the film captures the darkest side of this death culture. Wojnarowicz clearly describes AIDS as a plague in one of his poems, "Last Night," and, like Kramer, holds the American government "responsible for my death."[49] He believes that the Reagan administration's silence for eight years will result in his eventual death from AIDS (Wojnarowicz died two years after the film's release). As this poet's rage heightens, he calls America "this killing machine" and feels that increments of "rage" replace the loss of every one of his T cells.[50] His anger grows as his body is defeated by the virus. And he takes pleasure in fantasizing about how his dead body could be dropped on the front steps of the White House in order to provoke a reaction other than silence to this disease.

Yet the most extreme reaction to the discrimination accompanying AIDS is the raw and disturbing opening scene of Praunheim's film. We are drawn into a kitchen with a belligerent man talking about his newly discovered AIDS diagnosis. He contemplates whether or not the disease is a result of "germ warfare or the CIA"—not uncommon ideas during this time—while he is at the same time upset by some Republicans who arrived at an AIDS demonstration proclaiming, "you people get AIDS because you deserve it."[51] This man has already pulled a gun out of one of his cabinets as he sternly talks to the camera. He does not believe people deserve AIDS nor does he want to suffer socially or physically from this disease. He certainly precludes any future maltreatment as a person perceived to have a plague by inserting the gun in his rectum and releasing the trigger. This artistic depiction of an extreme type of rage turned inward is a sad testimony to the detrimental effects of discrimination experienced by people with AIDS during the first decade of its emergence.

On a lighter note, the first half of the 1990s also witnessed hedonism again as a reaction to the disease. Abraham Verghese's short story, *Lilacs*, captures this reaction in the main character's partner. Bobby is near the end of his life. He has AIDS and has been in Boston for any treatment he can get at one clinic. As he thinks about when he met Primo in his youth at Myrtle Beach, he cannot help thinking about the trajectory of their relationship. Primo, who also had AIDS, was horrified at the sight of other patients at this clinic in Boston when they arrived. He fled and subsequently engaged in reckless behavior, initially in flying his private plane and then in his sex life.

Bobby saw Primo's unprotected promiscuity as "poisoning as many others as he could, as if it would ease his own pain."[52] Hedonistic behavior during epidemics perceived as plagues certainly seems to help the bystanders forget about the suffering and death they have seen and that they might face themselves. Bobby, however, primarily sees Primo as a Gaeten Dugas who murders others through sex.

By the end of 1993 in San Francisco, unprotected anal intercourse was increasing again after years of safe practices. The Health Department, according to a survey, reported that one in three gay men in this city were indulging in this practice. One journalist was skeptical, and so am I, that a lack of education about safe sex explained this surge of behavior again, primarily because San Francisco launched one of the earliest and most vigorous safe sex programs in America. Instead Jane Gross explains that this behavior may be attributed to many gay men feeling "numb" over the loss of so many friends and lovers and feeling hopeless about their own survival. Other men surveyed were actually jealous of "the attention showered on the sick and dying" and engaged in risky behavior in an effort to get sick.[53]

On the other hand, younger gay men in San Francisco engaged in risky sexual behavior because they felt that AIDS was "the plague of an older generation and not their own."[54] These younger men in 1993 did not witness what seemed like countless numbers of lovers and friends carried away by the disease. Some people with AIDS actually were living longer in the early 1990s thanks to the increasing availability of other antiretroviral medications and more effective treatments for opportunistic infections. But many still died from the disease, a fact that highlights the strain of denial in this hedonistic logic.

An extreme fear of contagion also persisted within this death culture surrounding AIDS. In David Leavitt's story *Gravity*, Theo moves back home with his mother because of his growing blindness from CMV—the cytomegalovirus in AIDS patients that attacks many organs, including the retina in the eyes—and his increasing dependency on his mother to administer his Ganciclovir infusions in the hopes of slowing this deteriorating process. Sylvia, his mother, takes him out daily in spite of "his thinness and cane," two of the characteristic signatures of AIDS in young people at this time.[55] Many people by the early 1990s assumed that anyone under the age of 50, especially men, with this appearance had AIDS. And many people avoided the "thin" people because of an extreme and irrational fear of contagion of AIDS through casual contact. When Theo and Sylvia enter a gift shop in order to buy an expensive and delicate crystal bowl for a cousin's engagement party during one of their daily jaunts out of the house, the owner of the shop and his assistant are so pleased to see Sylvia. They warmly greet her but when she introduces her son to the men, "they didn't offer to shake hands."[56] This guarded discrimination, this invisible barrier erected between the uninfected and the infected, made people with AIDS feel even more like plague carriers.

In *Philadelphia*, Andy's lawyer, Miller, may grow to understand how much discrimination people with AIDS, especially gay ones, have endured, but at first he contributes to it as a result of his extreme fear of contagion and homosexuals. When Andy enters Miller's office in order to ask him to defend him in his lawsuit against his employer, Miller is terrified of catching AIDS. His body language is guarded as he stares at every part of the desk the ill-looking Andy touches. As Andy explains his maltreatment by the law firm, Miller asks him if he was not obligated to tell his employer that he "had this dreaded, deadly, infectious disease?"[57] By the time this movie was released in 1993, Americans certainly knew AIDS was not transmitted casually, but emotionally many people were not able to react calmly in the presence of someone with it because of the plague-making that had generated so much hysteria for over a decade.

Miller does not accept Andy's case at this time. And he is so worried about infection with HIV from this office meeting that he visits his doctor that very same day. In spite of his doctor explaining to him rationally that HIV can only be transmitted by an exchange of bodily fluids, Miller still insists he could have contracted the disease from this contact of consultation. His fear is so strong he even refuses to have his blood drawn for HIV antibodies, his doctor's solution for allaying his fears. The mere possibility of being HIV positive would mean suffering the discrimination experienced by his client, Andy Beckett.

Apocalyptic statements made about the nature of AIDS during this time did not diminish these fearful reactions in the general public at all. The HBO movie of Shilts' *And the Band Played On* captured the essence of the book and, like Shilts, portrayed AIDS as a plague resulting from the slow response of the government, which led to the disease's spread. Yet at the movie's climax with the international scientific race for the discovery of the virus and the fame associated with it, AIDS is described as an *uber* plague. When Dr. Don Francis at the CDC notices that many AIDS patients do not even display symptoms of the illness, he proclaims that "all the plagues in the history of the world got squeezed into this one."[58] This description of AIDS would have us believe that it is the culmination of every extant and extinct infectious disease, including *Yersinia pestis*, even though by 1993, when this movie was made, almost 34,000 Americans in a population of 250 million had died from AIDS and 2.5 million were infected with HIV in a global population of 5.5 billion.[59]

One of our most renowned poets, Allen Ginsberg, contributes to this AIDS hysteria during his interview in *Silence=Death*. Ginsberg makes it clear that he does not have HIV, but declares instead that "the planet itself has AIDS."[60] He discusses ozone depletion and the greenhouse effect as symptomatic of an environmental deficiency acquired by the earth as a result of human abuse and waste. In essence, humans are the immunodeficiency virus for the earth. Albeit poetic license is granted to Ginsberg's metaphor of AIDS for the illnesses of the planet, but it may reveal more about the poet's own fear of getting AIDS, which is projected onto the environmental state of our earth. This is not to deny the ailing state of our global climate, but 20 years after Ginsberg's statement we are still here. This type of fatalism about AIDS results from its creation as a plague and in turn feeds the plague hysteria surrounding the disease.

Reactions of projected disdain to AIDS continued alongside of the fear in this period. Dr. Abraham Verghese in *My Own Country* looks back at his initial experience with AIDS patients in the 1980s when he was a medical intern and provides some insight into why this disdain, as I describe it, existed for the AIDS patient. He reminds us that the American medical establishment in the early 1980s experienced "unreal and unparalleled confidence, bordering on conceit" in regard to treating and even curing most diseases.[61] Verghese admits that although cancer remained the one "fear" of medical doctors, even some cancers were being cured at this time. The medical community's certainty over controlling the course and outcome of most diseases was shattered with the emergence of AIDS here in the United States. And it was not difficult to subconsciously project this disdain of the uncontrollability and unpredictability of AIDS onto the AIDS patient. The suspended delay in medicine's magic to effectively treat AIDS fed this disdain.

And people with AIDS felt it, a feeling Kushner explores in Roy Cohn's revelation as he lay dying from AIDS in his hospital bed. Ethel Rosenberg's ghost often haunts Roy and at this moment in Act III of the drama she revels in his extreme abdominal pain. Roy manages to tell her though that "the worst thing about being sick in America is you are booted out of the parade. Americans have no use for sick."[62] The possibility of exiting the limelight of respect as a powerful lawyer explained Roy's objection to even admitting his AIDS diagnosis. On his death bed, Roy feels the American disdain toward the sick in general, let alone the AIDS patient. The plague mentality surrounding AIDS produced even more of this disdain because plagues have traditionally been viewed as shocking and uncontrollable epidemiological events causing much suffering and death. How very un-American.

This fear and projected disdain continued to feed the scapegoating of people with AIDS, the ultimate discriminatory reaction to diseases labeled as plagues. The risk groups that were staunchly institutionalized early in the epidemic remained the primary targets of blame for this disease. Jamie Feldman recognizes that although the "naming of risk groups" helped to demystify the illness initially in terms of not thinking it just comes out of the blue, "the political and social consequences" of this naming were not really evaluated prior to the widespread usage of risk groups within medical communities and in society at large.[63]

Even in 1994, the focus in the media remained on naming risk groups for AIDS. One article saw AIDS matter-of-factly "as a global plague" while describing "highly promiscuous gay men and abusers of intravenous drugs" as "the portals of entry" for AIDS into the Unites States from Africa.[64] Instead of presenting *how* HIV was supposedly transmitted transatlantically, this journalist contributed to the American cultural fixation on *who* transmits it. The consequences of assigning responsibility to these two groups once again, while at the same time referring to AIDS as a plague and conjuring up all of the word's attendant meanings and reactions, are persistent political and social discrimination toward these groups.

At this time, Texas ranked fourth in the country, tied with New Jersey, for the most number of AIDS cases, yet funding for the disease "ranked among the lowest states."[65] This neglectful fact was not surprising considering that it was still illegal to engage in homosexual intercourse in this state. The perpetual assumption in our society that AIDS was a gay disease, in spite of nongays with the disease now garnering more media attention, continued to fuel political neglect of its victims. And the political atmosphere in the 1990s here did not exactly embrace gay rights. Our government did not lift the ban on gays serving in the military. More conservative factions in the United States preferred to keep gay men and women serving and protecting us silently until the ban was finally repealed in December 2010.

Social discrimination against people with AIDS is powerfully portrayed in the library scene in *Philadelphia*. Andy Beckett appears thin and is coughing as he researches AIDS discrimination cases in preparation for his defense in court since Miller has not accepted his case yet. As the librarian brings Andy tomes to review, he asks him if he would prefer to move away from the general chamber of the library to the more private research room. Andy understands, as does Miller, who fortuitously witnesses this attempt at isolation, that the librarian's ultimate concern is not with Andy's comfort but with the public space of the library where it is too uncomfortable to view the perceived plague victim.

In one of the volumes, Andy finds the most apt description of the librarian's attempt to isolate him, which in turn will support his own case of AIDS discrimination. "Social death precedes physical death" for the AIDS sufferer, he reads aloud to Miller after he joins him at his table.[66] Once the AIDS victim is publically suspected of having this illness, as Andy was in his job, erstwhile social acceptance, indeed one's own social identity, decays rapidly.

In court, as Miller uncovers the discriminatory nature of this induced social death, he gets to the heart of this discrimination for people like Andy. "This case is not about AIDS," he declares to the room, but "the general public's hatred, loathing, and fear of homosexuals."[67] I also think it is about the establishment and maintenance of gay men as the premiere risk group for a disease created as a plague, which in turn propelled this discrimination even more.

Scapegoating of drug users—the other big sanctioned risk group along with prostitutes by this time, whose drug use often accompanied their labor and led to an increased HIV infection rate—continued in the form of legalized discrimination. A law maker in Texas felt that funding any type of AIDS program was a waste of money. His solution instead was "that infected prostitutes and drug users should be killed."[68] If these groups had not been presented in the media and medical literature as primary vectors of AIDS, appalling proposals like this one would not have been made. If AIDS had been presented as a disease anyone could contract through unsafe sex and dirty needles, drug users and prostitutes may not have been scapegoated like this.

And this established risk group felt the blame for the disease. Iris De La Cruz was a former drug user and prostitute who became an emergency medical technician in New York City. She was in the unique position of experiencing firsthand how these classifications result in blame, and she witnessed how the medical community contributed to producing these feelings in AIDS victims. She tells us in a personal essay that she helped a patient with pneumonia, brought into the ER by her, by suctioning him in order to ease his respiratory distress because the staff was not attentive to his needs at all. She declares that "medical staff, on the whole, resented AIDS patients"—there goes that projected disdain again—because they felt "they were all faggots and dope fiends and deserved what they got."[69]

When Cruz developed AIDS, she internalized this blame. She says she "felt unclean," and commented that other newly diagnosed people were "made to feel dirty" also.[70] One of my newly diagnosed patients at this time, Carl, immediately took a shower upon arriving on our unit. Every time we looked for him throughout the shift in order to complete his admission paperwork and administer medication, he was nowhere to be found. The hallway shower perpetually ran that evening. I finally caught him coming out of the shower and asked him if everything was O.K. "Sure," he said. "Then why have you taken so many showers this evening?" I inquired. "I just feel like I can't get clean." People with AIDS did not just naturally feel dirty. I have taken care of just as many cancer patients without AIDS and not one of them has ever expressed such a feeling to me. People with AIDS, especially those who fell into the stigmatized risk groups, were *made* to feel dirty by a society that overwhelmingly thought that this disease was deserved. AIDS patients were made to feel like they carried the very mark of sin.

As we have seen before, not everyone viewed AIDS patients as plague carriers who deserved what they got. A resident and founding family member of the Fire Island Pines, Mrs. Taussig, invited people with AIDS, regardless of any supposed risk group they fell into, to stay with her at her beach homes every summer since the epidemic's inception. In spite of initial harassment from neighbors and even the police, who did not want to see these sick people in their summer oasis, Mrs. Taussig continued to invite them to her homes every summer. In the early 1990s, she even entertained the homeless with AIDS.[71]

And many of us in the medical profession viewed AIDS patients not as plague carriers, but rather as victims of a horrible disease that kidnapped so many of them from the prime of their lives. By the spring of 1994, however, I was exhausted. I had cared for AIDS patients solely for almost seven years and not one of them had survived. One night when I arrived on duty, our devoted night nursing assistant asked, "Gina, did you hear, Randy Shilts died today?" I had not. I spent the morning in class and the afternoon sleeping in order to make it through my 13-hour shift. "He died of AIDS," Darren said. I knew that I was leaving for graduate school in a few months anyway, but this announcement confirmed for me that it was time to take a break. Randy Shilts inspired me to work with AIDS patients, and his death signaled my own departure far away from all this death.

But before I left that unit, I thought that just maybe my fatigue from witnessing so much physical, emotional, and social suffering in my patients and fighting for their right to be treated with dignity and respect might have turned me a little cold, a little hardened to it all. This burnout, as we call it, happened to several nurses I knew who worked with cancer patients for many years. I realized that indeed I was tired but not inured to it all when I entered Jonathan's room during 4 A.M. rounds to make sure he was OK—that meant still breathing.

Jonathan's bed had a view of one of the most beautiful bridges in Manhattan that was always a beacon during the black nights for all of us. Jonathan was not in his bed but sitting on the bedside commode smoking a cigarette with the oxygen blaring through a tube in his nostrils. I gently reminded him that he could blow us to smithereens and quickly asked him which one he needed more. I turned the oxygen off. He asked me to sit down and talk even though he was having diarrhea. "I go so much," he explained, "if I didn't talk to people while taking a shit, I wouldn't talk to anyone at all." Jonathan had cryptosporidium, a devastating intestinal parasite in AIDS patients that can produce diarrheal episodes up to and surpassing 25 times per day. He also invited me to share a Peep with him, those sweet marshmallow chick-shaped treats. This night was the eve of Good Friday. Jonathan spoke in strong tones with no regrets. He had lost a lot—a partner to AIDS and his jewelry business. But he was thankful for the prematurely short life he did live.

After about 30 minutes, Jonathan stood up from the commode. By now I had restored his oxygen. He was on his way back to bed and I turned away while saying "good night." What I did not realize until I reached the door of his room was that although I had been talking and listening to him for awhile, I was not really looking at him. I guess that was part of my defense that I had built in order to ward off my own pain from their suffering. But at the doorway with one faint light on, I looked back to make sure Jonathan made it to bed. And I looked *at* him. I had seen *Schindler's List* just a few months before this night and I was struck by how much he looked like a resident of Auschwitz. I guess I never absorbed the recent record of his weight of 75 pounds with a six-foot frame. "My God," I thought while keeping my composure, the supposed gold standard of a good nurse, after all these years, "they still pierce my soul." Jonathan died on Easter morning.

PART IV

The Endurance of AIDS

CHAPTER 9

Reflections (1995–2000)

"Is this the AIDS class?" a student nervously asked as I walked into the room. These second-semester freshmen had no choice but to register for a writing and literature class and I did not want to advertise ahead of time that the subject of this course was AIDS. My selection of the books for the class, however, was more revealing than I intended. On the university bookshelves, *And the Band Played On* and *Inventing the AIDS Virus* lay in waiting as required reading for them.

This class that I developed and taught for the spring 1999 semester was really the first time I began to open up about my experience of caring for AIDS patients during the worst years of the epidemic. I chose the following quote from Camus' novel to frame my course that would explore whether or not AIDS was a plague (the seeds of this book, it turns out): "At the beginning of a pestilence and when it ends, there's always a propensity for rhetoric. It is in the thick of a calamity that one gets hardened to the truth—in other words, to silence."[1] Although I walked into class on the first day fairly confident that AIDS was not a plague, in terms of it being a highly infectious disease like bubonic plague or a deserved one for some sin committed, I had to face the fact that personally I had a lot to say about AIDS when I began to care for these patients in the mid-1980s and a lot to say when I stopped taking care of them full time. But in the thick of this calamity—say from 1988 through 1994—there was an awful lot I did not say, really could not say. I only spoke superficially to family and friends about Cisco, Lenny, Larry, Kimberly, and Stephanie, for example, during the time I actually cared for them. It turns out my emotions were too raw and I unwittingly suppressed them. The physical suffering my patients endured and equally the psychological suffering that accompanied the disease rendered me hardened to the truth.

One student asked me, "Why did you choose this topic?" That was an easy one. I had a professional nursing background in AIDS and an academic one in medieval literature and history that focused on bubonic plague. Another student asked, "Why do homosexuals contract this disease?" That was a bit harder. Even by 1999, AIDS did not shake its connotation as a gay disease in the popular imagination. In order to learn more about my students' pre-conceptions about the disease, I asked them to respond in writing to the question: "What do you think of when you hear the word AIDS?" We shared their responses during the next class.

Mainly these young adults felt fear—some of them expressed downright panic—about contracting the disease, primarily because there was no cure for it and because they thought AIDS was a death sentence. None of them really knew anything about the new drug combination therapy that had been avail-able for four years at this point and actually held back the arm of death. They carried the effects of plague-making in their emotional worlds. For them, AIDS was a highly infectious disease that primarily affected gays and swept the nation, leaving tons of corpses in its path with no end in sight.

In reality, during this time there were new discoveries regarding AIDS that ended up delivering a great deal of hope. Perhaps the plague-making would finally stop. After all, by 1997, "AIDS was no longer one of the ten major causes of death in the United States."[2] The drop in the number of deaths now seemed to be inversely proportional to the rise in the number of people taking the new antiretroviral drugs.

Prior to 1995, we had AZT as the sole antiretroviral medication. It inhib-ited the reverse transcriptase enzyme that is responsible for transcribing HIV-RNA to DNA; stopping the enzyme's activity theoretically meant stop-ping the virus from reproducing. But clinical trials performed around this time provided other antiretrovirals (ARVs) such as ddI (Didanosine), which I remember administering when it was still in powder form for liquid dissolution on our AIDS unit as 1994 opened. During this year, several pharmaceutical companies also sponsored clinical trials that would offer com-binations of ARVs to participants with the main goal of quickly receiving FDA approval so that these treatments would be available to everyone with HIV/AIDS. Drug combinations such as AZT, ddI, 3TC, Nevarapine, and the very first protease inhibitor, Saquinavir, that blocked a different enzyme needed for viral replication, were administered with the intent of stopping the virus from reproducing at different stages. Like combination chemotherapy agents given to cancer patients in order to arrest the cancer cell in its different phases of division, the era of HAART (highly active antiretroviral therapy) had arrived for AIDS patients.[3]

By 1996, some European reports revealed success with these combina-tion regimens. In one report, 33 patients took AZT, 3TC, and Ritonavir, yet another new protease inhibitor, and after six months 15 patients had undetectable viral levels in their blood. Granted, this cohort of patients was not sufficient to prove efficacy in treatment for everyone with AIDS because the next 33 patients taking these drugs might not achieve the same response, but 15 more patients than ever before these drugs existed achieved success. Another study in British Columbia released encouraging results also with undetectable HIV levels in patients who took AZT, 3TC, and Nevarapine.[4]

Today, the different classes of ARVs and the single and combination drugs available are dizzying, to say the least. There are at least 30 FDA-approved single and combination drugs to treat HIV infection. But even in the mid-1990s, only 15 years after the first AIDS cases were reported in the United States, people with the disease had substantial treatment options. Some people felt like a new era in the AIDS epidemic had arrived. Andrew Sullivan, for example, announced near the end of 1995 that "medical science has turned a corner on effective treatment of AIDS and HIV," especially since six ARVs were available to everyone who needed them. Sullivan presciently commented that HIV is now being treated "as a chronic but manageable condition."[5] Granted, not everyone in 1995 or since then can tolerate the side-effects of these drugs. In early 1994, one of my patients taking ddI developed such profound numbness and tingling in his feet that he asked me to dump the medication down his drain one night. In addition, the new drugs were simply not effective in driving down the level of HIV, measured as HIV-RNA copies and referred to as the viral load, in some people who took them. According to one journalist in 1997, "between 10 and 30 percent of those who take the grueling course of new AIDS medications fail to respond."[6]

Yet by the late 1990s, the days of people dying after their first or second bout of PCP or uncontrollably wasting away to nothing were becoming distant nightmares of the illness. As the new drugs slowed down the virus, the immune system was less compromised and many people could live somewhat normal lives outside of hospital rooms. There was hope.

Other HIV cellular discoveries at this time fueled this hope about controlling the disease even more. Some American scientists studied close to 2,000 people at risk for contracting HIV—that meant all of the so-called risk groups—and they observed that 600 of those exposed to HIV never became infected with it.[7] In 1990, I cared for Tom, whose partner was absolutely flabbergasted that he never became HIV positive. He said they had countless numbers of unprotected sexual encounters before anyone knew about AIDS, and even though they tried to have safe sex after Tom was diagnosed, they were not always successful. And yet this man escaped infection.

Scientists discovered a genetic mutation that rendered one in 100 whites to have complete immunity to HIV infection and one in five whites to have slow progression to AIDS after infection with HIV in comparison with people without the mutation who did not develop any immunity.[8] The CCR5-Δ32 mutation alters the CCR5 co-receptor on white blood cells. Pathogens, like HIV, need a door to enter a cell and CCR5 is one such door. But if the CCR5 receptor door is defective, it cannot open and allow HIV inside. These scientists thought that an infectious disease approximately 700 years ago gave rise to this co-receptor mutation. Their disease candidate was *Yersinia pestis* because this bacillus also enters white blood cells through CCR5. If this mutation arose during the fourteenth-century bubonic outbreak across Europe, it would have conferred immunity to the disease in many people and allowed others to suffer a less lethal infection.[9]

It is indeed ironic that a disease traditionally viewed as the deadliest plague of the past may have played a major role in curtailing the disease that so many Americans have viewed as the modern plague. Furthermore, the discovery of this genetic mutation in the late 1990s led to the creation of another class of ARVs, the entry inhibitors that block HIV from entering the CCR5 co-receptor on white blood cells, and to the discovery of other cellular doors for AIDS—namely the CXCR4 co-receptor on white blood cells. These scientific discoveries about a disease consistently labeled as a plague since its emergence generated hope for controlling it.

Artistic works captured and contributed to this growing sense of hope that steadily began to surpass despair as a reaction to AIDS during the dawn of this HAART era. Hope has been a common reaction in periods following disease outbreaks in general and especially in those viewed as plagues. For instance, as the number of plague cases decreased in Oran and the city began to open its gates to the outside world, Albert Camus' narrator, Dr. Rieux, observes that "once the faintest stirring of hope became possible, the dominion of the plague was ended."[10] The hope revealed in some American art in the mid-to-late 1990s indicated that the dominion of AIDS as a plague started to abate.

There is a sense of optimism felt by those people with the disease, or directly affected by it, expressed most clearly for the first time since the epidemic emerged. In Adam Klein's short story *Keloid*, the reader experiences a postapocalyptic world featuring gay men in San Francisco. The narrator Adam thinks, as he sits next to Alan whom he has just met in a bar, that in earlier years he had to leave this city "in an effort to get away from AIDS," really to get away from all of the death.[11] Adam watched so many of his friends suffer and die from AIDS. But this is not the tenor of the city now.

In spite of Adam's former drug addiction, he did not become HIV positive and he has been in recovery for almost one year. On the other hand, Alan is HIV positive and taking at least one ARV. Alan, an AIDS psychobiologist, often picks up men in bars when he travels to conferences, like the AIDS one he will be presenting at in San Francisco. Finding a sexual mate in a bar is still a reality and so is having sex in a public place, but the perception of these commonplace pre-AIDS activities has changed. Adam, for instance, talking to Alan and glancing at two men having sex in the back of the bar, no longer sees public sex "as celebratory or radical" like he used to see it.[12]

More private sexual habits have changed as well in the aftermath of the worst years of the AIDS epidemic. Adam and Alan do not openly exchange bodily fluids when they have sex later back at Adam's apartment. Adam wants to stay negative and so he treats everyone as if they are HIV positive. Although Alan has not revealed his HIV status to Adam at this point, he protects him from any contact with his own semen during their rendezvous. "We made love like survivors, without the fears and petty encumbrances that might have made us afraid of deep kisses," Adam explains.[13] In 1995, when this story was published, these two men did not perceive themselves to be victims of AIDS. Adam is not even HIV positive and Alan seems fairly healthy and strong on the AZT he takes. Both men knew that viral transmission would not occur through passionate kissing; plus they do not exchange any fluids. The days of dismal reactions to AIDS seemed to be lifting.

In Jonathan Larson's successful Broadway musical, *Rent*, originally performed in 1996, AIDS has been absorbed into the American psyche, or at least the New York City one, primarily as a disease that one can live with. This world of struggling artists on Manhattan's lower East Side includes people with and without AIDS living together without fear like Roger and Mark; people with AIDS finding love like Tom Collins and Angel and eventually Roger and Mimi; and AZT sprinkling many of the scenes as several of the characters take it and it is sold as a commodity in St. Mark's Place alongside other wares.[14]

There are remnants of beliefs about AIDS from the primary plague-making years. Roger, a musician who contracted AIDS from his former girlfriend who killed herself when she found out about her diagnosis, sees AIDS as a death sentence and a barrier to any new relationship. When Mark tries to understand why Roger will not ask out Mimi, a young, attractive girl who lives beneath them in their tenement building and is obviously interested in him, Roger explains that he would rather go out to eat because it is "the one vice left—when you're dead meat."[15] Roger definitely feels like people with AIDS did in the pre-HAART era. He equally feels a sense of urgency about composing his music before HIV overtakes his body.[16]

Roger and Mimi are also quite reluctant to reveal their respective HIV positive status to each other, a reticence resulting from cultural perceptions that AIDS is a plague. One of their sung refrains to each other is "I should tell you" as they move closer and closer to each other and cannot fight their physical attraction.[17] Each of them fears the rejection that has traditionally been a response to the HIV carrier. Neither one of them ever garners the courage to openly admit their viral status; rather they discover it by accident later when their beepers alarm to remind them it is time to take their AZT.

Different attitudes about AIDS in this drug treatment era, however, do actually gain dominance on this musical stage. Angel and Tom Collins are forthright about the disease they each carry when they first meet. Angel tells Tom that she carries the virus when she finds him beaten up on the street sidewalk outside of Roger and Mark's apartment building. Tom admits he also has it.[18] Subsequently they become a happy couple. Although Angel eventually dies from AIDS, an unfortunate reminder that the virus still can kill, she is the only character with the disease who perishes; plus she has been the love of Tom's life.

Hope begins to replace despair in this artistic depiction of people living with AIDS. The support group for people with the disease is called "'Life Support' Group."[19] Every member of this group has dealt with the death of a loved one from AIDS and many of them have the disease themselves but their focus is on the present, not the past. They want to find happiness in the present moment without fear of the future or regret of the past.

All of the characters meet after Maureen's performance art event at an eponymously hopeful hangout, the "Life Café."[20] Here, Mimi and Roger embrace after they discover that they share a mutual dependence on AZT. All of the characters embrace their bohemian life as artists and as people living with or dealing with AIDS. Everyone proclaims their commitment to combating AIDS when they collectively sing, "Actual Reality—ACT UP—Fight AIDS."[21] Indeed there was hope now for living with AIDS. This hope would not have been possible without the anger that inspired Larry Kramer and other activists who tirelessly urged scientists to offer better treatment options.

A few years later, Michael Cunningham's *The Hours* dealt in part with this transitional phase of reactions to AIDS as a plague. Cunningham's novel is a modern-day version of Virginia Woolf's 1925 novel, *Mrs. Dalloway*. Woolf's narrative takes place over 24 hours and focuses mainly on Clarissa Dalloway's thoughts, feelings, and memories as she moves about London in her efforts to prepare for a party that evening. Cunningham's novel shifts between Virginia Woolf living outside of London at the time she was writing her novel; Clarissa Vaughn, his version of Clarissa Dalloway who lives in 1990s New York City; and Mrs. Brown, a post–World War II housewife who is reading *Mrs. Dalloway* in an attempt to escape the traditional role of wife and mother that has been imposed upon her by American society at that time.

Cunningham's character Richard embodies a despairing response to AIDS. Richard is Clarissa Vaughn's oldest friend and lover, and the son of Mrs. Brown. He is also the mirror for Woolf's shell-shocked Septimus Smith, who commits suicide in her novel. Clarissa is throwing a party of her own this evening in New York City for Richard, whose talent as a poet has earned him a prestigious literary award. But Richard's despair over his illness pervades his vision of this bestowed award. He refuses to believe that he received the prize based on the merit of his work; rather he thinks, "I got a prize for having AIDS and going nuts and being brave about it."[22] Richard has absolutely no hope about his future in general. In spite of the table-full of medications he takes, he is dying. Clarissa explains to one of Richard's former lovers who is in town for his party, "I'm afraid he was a little too far gone for the protease inhibitors to help him the way they're helping some people."[23] His HIV dementia unfortunately developed before this class of drugs was available in the mid-1990s. Now none of his ARVs can reverse the viral damage to his body and especially to his brain. Before Richard kills himself by jumping out of his window when Clarissa arrives at his dingy apartment to chauffer him to his ceremony and party, he desperately utters, "I'm so sick."[24]

Hope for people with AIDS, however, has a place in Cunningham's book. Those who were able to receive HAART before too much damage was done to their systems live more normal lives instead of a life of isolation that Richard lived in his apartment. When Clarissa begins her day of chores leading up to the party, she sees a mutual friend of theirs, Walter Hardy, whose lover has been suffering from AIDS. But Evan is "feeling so much better on this new cocktail" and wants to go out dancing tonight, according to Walter. Prior to HAART, this seemingly normal activity was impossible for Evan. Walter assures Clarissa that not only is dancing not too strenuous for Evan but "he just wants to be out in the world again."[25] And he can be now.

During this period, real people also experienced hope about living social lives again in spite of their AIDS diagnosis. John Kelly's vignette of Edward, an AIDS clinical trials participant in the mid-1990s whom Kelly follows through treatment, illustrates the move from a state of despair to one of hope. Edward's friend Corky comments on how Edward began to isolate himself in the early 1990s when he had been HIV positive for a few years. Then Edward felt like "HIV neuters you," and he gave up thinking about any intimate relationship.[26] But when a clinical trial opened in New York City with a new protease inhibitor (Indinivar) being tested, Edward wanted to enter it. Not only was he eligible for the study—an impressive accomplishment for anyone due to the strict entry criteria—but he ended up receiving the combination of drugs that did not include placebos. And he did well on these drugs. After four years of celibacy, he also started to think about a relationship again.

A highly regarded scholar whom I cared for in 1990 died from lymphoma, according to his obituary, with no mention of the AIDS that actually killed him. The atmosphere was changing though. There was hope now that discrimination against people with AIDS was dissipating right along with all of that despair. By 1995, more and more obituaries were revealing the cause of death as AIDS and not as the colloquial "long illness." Families of those who died from AIDS were less fearful about others' reactions to this publically stated cause of death. A December 30, 1995, obituary, for example, quoted the deceased artist's mother: "the cause [of death] was AIDS."[27] And Prior in *Angels in America* captured this breakthrough on the silence surrounding death from AIDS when he announces proudly at the play's conclusion, "we won't die secret deaths anymore."[28]

Discrimination against people living with AIDS still existed, but at least legal ramifications for it were becoming a reality. In 1996, a cruise line had to award $90,000 to a man whose job offer they retracted when he tested positive for HIV. Dolphin Cruise Line Inc. attempted to justify this action by claiming the HIV positive job candidate "would pose a significant risk of harm to himself and others because of his condition."[29] The cruise line's view of AIDS was mired in plague-making. Company officials saw the disease as a highly infectious one that could be spread by casual contact. But the Miami Office of the Equal Opportunity Commission (EOC), which filed the lawsuit on behalf of the plaintiff, would not tolerate this discriminatory view. The EOC won the suit based on the fact that AIDS had been deemed a disability, and furthermore employment should not be contingent upon one's HIV status, especially in jobs where fluid exchange was highly unlikely. This commission broke out of a plague mentality at a time when more and more people were living much longer with HIV and AIDS.

The hope of living with AIDS propelled some writers to see the disease as actually entering a post-plague era. Andrew Sullivan refers to AIDS de facto as a plague in his 1996 piece, "When Plagues End," because it had killed so many of his friends and acquaintances. He also admits that when he became HIV positive, he could not help feeling like he was responsible for the illness, a feeling he relates to his own discomfort with being gay. "I instinctively interpreted," he says, "this illness as something that I deserved."[30] This sense of disease as punishment is not "instinctive" in the least but a result of our society's construction of AIDS as a plague, in particular as a disease wielded upon people for what has been deemed a socially unacceptable sexual orientation.

The point of Sullivan's article, however, is that "this plague is over," even though many scientists and medical doctors did not see it that way. Sullivan saw that AIDS "no longer signifies death" and that we were on the horizon of a post-plague era.[31] The new ARVs at least provided the possibility of living with the disease "as a manageable, chronic condition"—the way Andrew Jacobs also describes it a few months after Sullivan's article. Jacobs actually highlights people with AIDS, however, who cannot revel in this view: the 10–30 percent of people who have failed the new treatment and felt even more miserable when they heard that the plague was behind us.[32] Despair was still extant.

Like these people with AIDS who have not responded to treatment, there were other writers, including scientists, who, unlike Sullivan, were not convinced that a new era had arrived in the United States or in the world at large. These writers instead focused on the continual rise in the number of deaths from the disease, treatments that did not cure let alone were simply not effective for some people, and the disease's reach across the globe.

By the late 1990s, some 400,000 people had died from AIDS in America alone.[33] It was also the "leading cause of death" among American blacks between the ages of 25 and 49.[34] Ten years earlier, the number of deaths from the disease in the United States was 50,000. This eightfold increase, in addition to our country being only in the infancy of an effective treatment era for AIDS, accounts for a persistent view of AIDS as a plague. James Giblin's *When Plague Strikes* would have impressed upon a younger reader in 1995 when it was published that AIDS has a place in a long lineage of plagues. Although the book may not have had a substantial impact on an adult audience, it was written with historical accuracy. Yet Giblin actually presents AIDS as worse than bubonic disease and smallpox because "it has by no means been brought under control."[35] Of course by the mid-1990s, the smallpox vaccine had brought this disease under control and an arsenal of effective antibiotics did the same for bubonic disease. Combination drug therapy had only been approved for widespread usage by people with AIDS and its proven efficacy was in a state of suspension until more time passed.

Immunobiologist Michael B. Oldstone referred to AIDS as "a plague as bad as any ever known" in his book on different infectious diseases written a few years after Giblin's book.[36] By now, some time had passed for a better assessment of the efficacy of combination therapy. Oldstone does not imply that AIDS is a plague because it is a deserved punishment from a divine source for some sinful behavior, rather it is one because "40 million individuals are already infected" and there is no cure for it.[37] Although this scientist acknowledges the advent of HAART, he dismisses its efficacy for the majority of people living with HIV/AIDS. His failure rates for HAART corroborate with Jacobs' figure of 10–30 percent, but he focuses solely on this minority who fail treatment, which has the effect of keeping the course of AIDS quite dismal. "Even with present combination therapy," he points out, "nearly a quarter of treated individuals are not helped."[38] Perhaps a focus on the three quarters of treated people who *are* helped would have altered Oldstone's view of AIDS as a hopeless diagnosis with a high mortality rate. It was hard, however, to escape the plague mentality that had cloaked America for so long.

Other writers focused on the global impact of AIDS, which explains why they viewed it as a plague. Biologist Paul W. Ewald described AIDS in his 2000 book on infectious diseases as "a new kind of pandemic plague."[39] According to scientific lore, AIDS emerged on the African continent after it was transmitted to humans by some other primate (probably the African green monkey) and eventually made its way around the globe. A local emergence of a disease resulting in a global spread qualifies AIDS as a new plague for Ewald. Science journalist Gina Kolata also sees AIDS as a plague for this reason. She admits that AIDS "is much less contagious" than bubonic plague but describes it as "another plague that has ravaged the world."[40] And an anonymous *New York Times* article in early 2000 not only presents AIDS as a "global plague" because of its geographical impact and the "tens of millions" infected with it, but also notes that "there is still no cure and no vaccine."[41] People living in poorer countries than the United States notably could not afford the $15,000 annual expenditure required for combination therapy. And without this treatment, death is practically inevitable, as it was before this era.

The plague-making during this period stemmed from the focus on AIDS as a highly infectious disease with a high mortality rate. National and international statistics for those infected with HIV and dead from AIDS support this focus. But there is an alternative one that circumvents this plague view. The number of AIDS deaths in the United States at this time was admittedly worrisome, but the 400,000 dead in a U.S. population of approximately 270 million in 1999 qualifies the death rate from AIDS as a quite small percentage (less than 1 percent) of the resident population. This percentage does not suggest that AIDS is a highly infectious disease with a high mortality rate. Bubonic disease killed more than half of the entire European population within a few years during its devastating visit in the fourteenth century. It seems that hyperbole still accompanied discussions of AIDS as the twentieth century closed. Although these writers endorsed a viral cause of AIDS and not a divine one, continuing to discuss AIDS as a plague kept the door open for others to find human causes for it. This search always seems to lead to some degree of scapegoating.

Microbiologist Peter Duesberg joined the few scientists, like Robert Root-Bernstein, who questioned the viral cause of AIDS. It would have been more difficult to publically question this if AIDS simply had been accepted much earlier in American society as a new infectious disease that could be controlled with practices that dissuaded the transmission of HIV, such as using condoms during any sexual intercourse and using clean needles when injecting recreational drugs, instead of as an uncontrollable disease that was deserved for certain behaviors considered taboo in American society. Irrational thinking about the disease would have been rejected prima facie by 1995 if it had not been made into a plague.

Viewing AIDS as a plague while ignoring the promise of new drug therapies continued to inspire searches for causes other than the viral one, which had been firmly established and universally accepted by the medical community and even the lay community at large well before the 1990s. Dr. Karry B. Mullis' "Foreword" to Duesberg's *Inventing the AIDS Virus* illustrates some of the long-term effects of plague-making a disease. Mullis is a Nobel laureate in chemistry for the invention of the PCR test (Polymerase Chain Reaction) that ironically would be used by AIDS scientists a few years after her discovery to measure the amount of HIV-RNA in the blood, popularly referred to as the viral load test. Without her discovery we could not measure this viral load, a measurement doctors have depended on since the mid-1990s in order to guide ARV treatment decisions. If the viral load rises in any given person, clinicians add and subtract different drugs from the combination regimen in an effort to drive down the level of HIV in the blood.

Mullis is suspicious that there was no "*original* paper where somebody showed that HIV caused AIDS."[42] She wonders why we do not have the definitive "origins" for "a disease increasingly regarded as a twentieth century Black Plague."[43] It may be difficult to understand why a Nobel Prize–winning chemist has not accepted Luc Montagnier's and Robert Gallo's co-discovery of HIV as the cause of AIDS a decade before she wrote this piece, like it is for me. Both scientists present the history of their respective laboratory discoveries of HIV in their joint article "AIDS in 1988," which was published in *Scientific American*. They stated clearly that "contributions from our laboratories—in roughly equal proportions—have determined that the cause of AIDS is a new human retrovirus." They confidently proclaim "that HIV is the cause of AIDS is by now firmly established."[44] Mullis does not acknowledge this paper and concludes her "Foreword" by encouraging us to read Duesberg's book because "the HIV/AIDS hypothesis is one hell of a mistake."[45] Whether or not Mullis' friendship with Duesberg clouded her own scientific judgment regarding the cause of AIDS is anyone's guess, but her rejection of the viral cause coupled with her references to the disease as a modern plague ignites the atmosphere for Duesberg's own causation theory.

First and foremost, Duesberg does not believe that HIV causes AIDS based on his assumption that the virus does not fulfill Koch's postulates (Root-Bernstein's theory). He also believes that AIDS is not infectious because it has not spread beyond the original risk groups, primarily gays and IVDUs.[46] Root-Bernstein's rejection of HIV/AIDS fulfilling Koch's postulates was a bit shortsighted, as I mentioned before, and the same can be said for Duesberg's similar claim. But Duesberg's claim that AIDS is not infectious is a downright dangerous message for laypeople, as was Root-Bernstein's proposal that AIDS does not infect "healthy" people. Furthermore, Duesberg's view that AIDS has not left the gay male or IVDU communities keeps the onus of burden for the disease solely on these people.

Duesberg believes that AIDS has been a fabrication by the medical community. According to him, cervical cancer was only added to the AIDS surveillance definition in 1993 by the CDC in order "to increase the number of female AIDS patients" and "create an illusion" that the disease was "spreading into the heterosexual population."[47] Gina Corea would not be happy with this statement, nor would all of the women out there who fought for recognition of this cancer, in the presence of HIV, to be accepted as an AIDS-defining illness. Cervical cancer, however, is not the only disease that women with HIV experienced. Like my patients Kimberly and Stephanie, women with HIV contracted diseases other than cervical cancer. This cancer alone was not driving up the female AIDS population. The CDC's November 1995 *MMWR* noted that the percentage of female AIDS cases increased from "8 percent of cases reported during 1981–1987 to 18 percent during 1993–October 1995."[48] Based on what I saw as an AIDS nurse in New York City in the early 1990s, this increase in females with AIDS was a reality. Furthermore, the CDC report demonstrated a 7 percent increase in "heterosexual transmission" in the absence of drug use during the same time period.[49]

Instead of accepting a rise in the number of females and other heterosexuals with AIDS, Duesberg's ultimate goal is to support the question: "What if drugs caused AIDS?"[50] This is fair enough to ask, but when he further claims that "recreational drugs have never left the major AIDS risk groups, i.e., male homosexuals and intravenous drug users," we have entered the familiar territory of scapegoating.[51] There are plenty of gay men who do not use any recreational drugs and plenty of straight people who do.

Duesberg discusses drugs like cocaine and amphetamines lowering the immune system and leading to any one of the diseases considered an AIDS-defining diagnosis. He even claims at one point that there are more than 4,000 cases of people dying from diseases that qualify as AIDS and they are HIV negative, but he only references his own work for this statistic.[52] Most importantly, he misunderstands the fact that people do not die of AIDS if they are HIV negative. An AIDS diagnosis is only made in the presence of the human immunodeficiency virus. The medical community does not consider anyone to have AIDS, no matter what disease the person has on the AIDS surveillance list, if that person is HIV negative. I am caring for someone right now in the summer of 2010 who has PCP and is HIV negative. This pneumonia is considered a complication of immunosuppression stemming from his non-Hodgkin's lymphoma diagnosis and chemotherapy treatment.

The British journalist Edward Hooper did not deny that HIV is the cause of AIDS during this time, but he blames humans for its spread, in particular the scientific community that produced the OPV (oral polio vaccine) in the 1950s. He sees these scientists as responsible for introducing HIV, albeit unwittingly, into the human population, and he implicates the gay male community in the United States in the process of trying to prove his theory.

Hooper's *The River* probably should not be discussed in the same context as Duesberg's work. Hooper actually interviewed Duesberg in 1990 and was not convinced by his drug causality theory, and was even less impressed by the California scientist's reluctance to fulfill his own offer to inject himself with HIV in order to prove that it does not cause AIDS. Hooper saw Duesberg as belonging to "those conspiracy theorists who believe that we are kept in the dark about the 'true nature of AIDS.' "[53] Yet Hooper's own work falls within this conspiracy realm.

Hooper was attracted to theories that linked the origin of HIV to the production of the OPV in the 1950s. One of the vaccine discoverers, Dr. Albert Sabin, accused another one, Dr. Hilary Koprowski, of unintentionally contaminating some lots of the polio vaccine with a simian virus (SV40). Many scientists have considered this simian virus in the monkey population to be a possible precursor of HIV.[54] Hooper's entire tome is devoted to searching for evidence that proved that these original oral polio vaccines contained a simian viral contaminant that children swallowed—the route of vaccine administration—in the Congo region of Africa. Supposedly, this simian virus eventually became HIV and the virus spread to other humans from this original source. Never mind that Sabin said if there was an HIV precursor viral contaminant, it would not have survived the swallowing process. Gastric enzymes and acid render HIV impotent. Never mind that a special scientific committee was convened in October 1992 that addressed this contamination theory and concluded that "the probability of the AIDS epidemic having been started by the inadvertent inoculation of an unknown HIV precursor into African children during the 1957 polio virus vaccine trials [was] extremely low."[55] Hooper dogmatically searches for this connection between OPV and the introduction of HIV into humans in spite of prominent scientists' definitive rejection of the connection.

There is no scientific validity for Hooper's argument that OPV administered in the Congo was the ultimate source of HIV in humans. His thesis, however, warrants consideration in terms of its influence on how the general public might view AIDS. He tells his readers that he wants them to consider "the very real possibility that humans have unwittingly unleashed this dreadful epidemic upon themselves."[56] Hooper believes the polio vaccine discoverers did not intend to transmit a deadly virus in their quest to eradicate polio globally, but nonetheless he blames AIDS on a human source. The offering of a human source for diseases is a salient characteristic of plague-making, even though he does not call AIDS a plague.

The gay male community, unfortunately, is never too far from reach when it comes to assigning human blame for AIDS. At one point, Hooper presents an attorney's theory on one major mode of HIV's introduction into America: Gay men in the 1970s took the OPV in an effort to fight off herpes infections. Hooper does not endorse this theory as a provable one but believes that it "made an important contribution to the origins debate" of HIV.[57] It certainly contributes to the already popular notion in the United States that the origin of this disease was gay men. And Hooper's logic suggests that just maybe if gay men did not have all that sex and contract herpes, they would not have used a vaccine that supposedly carried the viral precursor of HIV. Then we would not have AIDS in this country.

As Hooper examines the spread of AIDS in the United States by the end of his book, he utters a quite familiar plague refrain: "the virus is moving *from* its original target group, gay men, *to* the general population."[58] Gay men were still presented here as giving birth to this epidemic and as isolated members of the wider society. They were still held responsible for the spread of this disease to everyone else. Certainly Hooper's primary scapegoat for AIDS was the polio vaccine scientists, but gay men cannot step into the shade of plague-making blame.

Even by the 1990s, the gay male in American society was still treated with disdain because early on he had been assigned the status of primary vector of AIDS. Jeanette Farrell, in her book on infectious diseases, discusses an incident at the White House in 1995 that epitomizes this treatment of them. Some gay political leaders were invited there—an invitation that at least indicated some acceptance of the gay community by the president—but the Secret Service donned rubber gloves to perform the customary inspection of their belongings.[59] These men were still viewed as the bearers of a plague that could be contracted easily through touch.

Gay males were also treated with disdain by some members of the African American community, especially when the focus was on AIDS. This community's fear of being blamed by the white community for AIDS coupled with their reluctance to openly discuss sexuality in general influenced their view of gay men. Thomas Glave's 1997 short story, *The Final Inning*, through its stream of consciousness narrative technique reveals one black community's discriminatory reactions to AIDS. Duane has died of AIDS and the reader is made privy to the postfuneral world of family and friends rehashing what they see as the mortifying event at Duane's funeral. Jimmy cared for Duane and stood up in the front of the church begging Duane's loved ones to just admit that he had AIDS and that he was gay. Jimmy feels like his own African American community is "killing us" because its members will not talk about AIDS or homosexuality.[60] Black gay men with AIDS felt socially isolated (a form of death) from their own families and friends who were unwilling for the most part to have these open conversations. The earlier Silence = Death movement at least influenced Jimmy's ability to stand up in front of his community and let them know the detrimental effects of their silence.

The collective voice of Duane's family and friends at the funeral is presented alongside of Jimmy's speech asking for openness. Their thoughts reveal familiar views of AIDS. "No my son ain't no homosexual no my cousin ain't no faggot," think Duane's mother and cousin as they listen to Jimmy.[61] One of Duane's aunts thinks, "no my nephew didn't have no damn AIDS the *devil's* disease."[62] For many of them, AIDS is evil because gay people get it.

At Tamara's house after the funeral, Jacquie's husband, Gregory, thinks about the effects of this community's denial of AIDS on Duane after Nicky admits that she was one of the only people with whom Duane felt comfortable enough to reveal his disease: "Didn't want nobody to know you had *it*."[63] Gregory understands that Duane's family and friends prefer not to even say the word and instead officially reference the disease as "it," a popular pronoun for AIDS throughout the 1980s and 1990s that still managed to evoke horror and judgment. And when Duane's family and friends actually had to face his diagnosis, they reach for the most popular scapegoat created in American culture at large. Gregory thinks, "when they heard you had it said yup serves his ass right cause you *know* he got it from hanging out with them nasty old white boys village faggots downtown too much."[64] The Lower West Side of Manhattan remains the wellspring of white gay men and AIDS, and, of course, Duane deserves *it* for being gay.

Plague-making is essential in the community Glave depicts for keeping its members "safe from the truth."[65] This is also Gregory's intent for his own family. The reader knows that Gregory is not only attracted to other men but secretly engages in sexual encounters with them. The *truth* is that there are gay people in the black community and the *truth* is that gay and straight black men and women get AIDS in the same ways as white, Asian, and Indian people do. Viewing AIDS as a plague that primarily strikes down white gay males is one way for this community to keep itself safe from the truth that this disease also affects it. The stigma that AIDS had acquired by the mid-to-late 1990s from being created as a plague kept gay black men like Duane semisilent about their disease and sexuality, and black men like Gregory completely silent about any sexual feelings for other men. Who could live openly with the possibility that one's very sex life would incur judgment from God in the form of AIDS?

People in many communities during this time still did not feel comfortable with others even thinking they had AIDS. In Wilmington, Delaware, for example, an HIV program in 1996 noticed that at least half of its patients who became HIV positive were not going to the hospital annex to receive care. The HIV program director explained that "there is still an amazing stigma associated with a diagnosis of HIV infection."[66] When this HIV program created satellites in non-medical facilities where patients could be treated and not suspected of having HIV as they walked through the doors, they showed up for their appointments.

It would be hard to deny that the last half decade of the twentieth century provided hope for people living with HIV and AIDS as a result of the new combination drug therapies. I care for patients today who were diagnosed during this era and are still alive because of these medications, whereas everyone I cared for in the pre-HAART era is not. Also, during the final years of the last century, overt and violent discrimination against people with this disease diminished considerably. Fewer people viewed AIDS as a disease that was readily contracted through touch or as a deserved punishment for sexual orientation and certain behaviors. But the plague-making that had occurred in our culture earlier, and the remnants of it that persisted, had been internalized by many communities and contributed to the silence that people living with HIV/AIDS chose as a response to their diagnosis as the twenty-first century arrived.

CHAPTER 10

Reticence (2001–2010)

Admittedly, I was more excited about the possibility of taking care of someone with anthrax when it was being distributed in the mail and ventilation systems in the D.C. area where I was living than I was about taking care of someone with newly diagnosed tuberculosis. After all, I had cared for countless numbers of young TB patients on the AIDS unit in New York City during the 1980s and 1990s.

But now it was December, 2001, and I was in Baltimore, Maryland, working a shift in a local hospital's pulmonary unit. It was actually one of my first visits to this city and I had no idea that TB was still so prevalent. My years in Pennsylvania between New York and Maryland shielded me from this reality. Nor did I realize that many people were still terrified to even face the possibility of an AIDS diagnosis. I thought that six years after the advent of all new drugs to treat HIV, anyone now dealing with this diagnosis would be a bit more accepting and hopeful than in 1985. At least I thought there would be more of a willingness to talk about HIV like my patient Mary who I was caring for at the far end of the hallway on this pulmonary unit. She knew every one of the 12 antiretroviral pills I gave her on evening medication rounds. She was forthcoming about her diagnosis and she felt lucky to be alive so many years after seroconverting.

But Daryl at the other end of the hallway felt a bit different. He also was quite sick. He was only 22 years old and had just returned home to Baltimore after living in Atlanta the last couple of years. I could not get his temperature to go down below 102 degrees Fahrenheit throughout my shift. This challenge felt familiar. He was just diagnosed with TB and the medications we were giving him had not squelched the bacillus yet. He was also being worked up for anal cancer—a cancer that was increasingly being seen in people with HIV who also carried HPV (the genital warts virus). But at this time the convergence of two viruses resulting in another cancer was not completely understood.

Daryl also was being worked up for AIDS in light of these other diseases that visited his body. His HIV test had been drawn the day before and the medical team was anxiously awaiting the results so that decisions could be made. I garbed up outside of his room and entered. He was scared. Scared because he never saw anyone's face. Scared because he did not understand why he felt so ill. Scared because he knew on some level what he was facing.

I gave him some of his medication for the tuberculosis shortly after I entered his room. "Will I get better?" he asked. I assured him that the TB could be tamed. Then I explained that we had to see if he was HIV positive or not in order to know how to prevent other infections in the future, including the TB. He was shocked. "You mean I have AIDS?" I knew he signed a consent form the day before for the test but I asked him if he remembered signing it. "Yes," he said, "but I didn't think I would have AIDS." It seemed like Daryl had no clue about the strong possibility of having AIDS, even though the medical team had prepared him, or just maybe this misunderstanding was being fed by something scarier. And so I engaged him in a conversation about how he ended up here in this Baltimore hospital.

Daryl told me he had moved to Atlanta about two years ago and was living with a "friend." This friend assured him that he did not mess around and Daryl wanted to believe him. He pretended that he did. He was just starting to realize and admit that Kevin may have endangered his own life by not wearing a condom during their sexual relations. I asked Daryl where Kevin was now and he said he was still in Atlanta. I asked him if Kevin knew he was sick. "He stopped answering my calls when I told him I was here," Daryl revealed.

It was bad enough that Daryl had to come to terms with his partner's infidelity and the very strong possibility that this was a factor in his illness now. But even worse was having to deal with his mother who forcefully made her presence known on the unit when she arrived. "Who's my son's nurse?" she bellowed at the nurse's station. Being the lucky candidate, I took her to the most private place I could find. She hovered over me in the kitchen. "Does my boy have AIDS?" I explained that the HIV test results were pending and then prepared her for the possibility that he did have it. But she was more concerned with how he might have contracted the virus. She continued, "Did that faggot he was living with in Atlanta give it to him? I'll kill him if he did."

This woman's anger over how her son might have gotten AIDS—his HIV test was positive—captures some of the African American community's reactions to male homosexuality and AIDS. Daryl's mother was openly gay herself but could not deal with her own son being gay or especially with the strong possibility that he acquired the disease through unprotected sex with a male partner. And Daryl could not speak openly with his mother about his AIDS diagnosis or his own sexual orientation. Reticence reigns as the AIDS sufferer's primary reaction to the disease even as a new century offers more treatment options.

The African American community exhibited this reaction to AIDS several decades after its appearance because the disease continued to be viewed as a plague in our country. Cathy Cohen, a professor of political science and African American studies at Yale University, explores the complex reasons underlying her community's slow and somewhat ineffective response to the AIDS epidemic while facilely calling it a "devastating plague."[1] Gil L. Robertson's Introduction to a powerful collection of essays from members of the black community who want to break the silence enveloping AIDS begins by calling the disease "this scourge." He explains, albeit tautologically, that this scourge of AIDS "has trampled on us like an unabated plague."[2] *AIDS*, *scourge*, and *plague* have become interchangeable terms.

Cohen and Robertson do not endorse, by any means, what I have argued are the effects of plague-making—primarily discrimination against the viral carriers. Both writers are actually attempting to persuade their communities to be open and vocal about this disease and other issues, such as poverty, drug abuse, and sexuality that intersect with its occurrence. Yet references to AIDS as a plague unintentionally contribute to the very reluctance of black communities to discuss AIDS.

Certainly proclaiming that "HIV and AIDS have literally become the black plague," as one African American journalist did near the end of 2005, does not abet a willingness to talk about AIDS.[3] In addition, this writer sees many of the problems in his community—namely "poverty, ignorance, illness, and violence"—as "self-inflicted."[4] The implication of this pronouncement is that these "self-inflicted" problems have also led to the "black plague" of AIDS within this community. These statements seem to drive us into the familiar territory of viewing AIDS as a deserved punishment for certain conditions that had already been blamed for causing past plagues, like poverty. The journalist's call for "changes in behavior" within the black community that could, as he sees it, "halt the self-destruction that is consuming so many black lives"[5] cannot be achieved if AIDS continues to be perceived as a plague that this community is inflicting upon itself. No one wants to think that his or her level of knowledge, social status, drug use, or sexual practices incurs punishment. If AIDS instead is presented as a preventable disease and not as a punishment, behaviors can be discussed in a nonjudgmental fashion and then changed.

Atlanta Gospel music director Byron Cage may call AIDS "a modern-day plague" in his essay because it has killed so many people in his community and has spread around the globe, yet he criticizes what I term the *plague-making blame* perpetuated by other writers.[6] Cage lambastes his own church for a mentality that has resulted in discrimination of people with AIDS. He reflects that "it is unfortunate that the black church has preached for many years that AIDS is a punishment for gay people."[7] Cage, like some gay writers throughout the epidemic, classifies AIDS as a plague because it has affected so many people in his own community and not because he thinks that his community deserves the disease. By the time Cage wrote his essay, the rate of HIV infection was actually more than eight times higher among blacks than whites in the 1 million people living with AIDS in the United States.[8]

Even when AIDS is not presented as a punishment for certain behaviors, the persistent reference to the disease as plague keeps alive perceptions of it as a highly contagious disease that should be feared. Robi Reed reveals in her essay, for example, that her Uncle Jimmy made a chicken dish that her family always loved to eat, but after he was diagnosed with HIV no one in the family would touch it.[9]

Even the mere suspicion of AIDS produces this fear of the plague victim in some black communities. Jacob Levenson highlights these communities affected by AIDS in rural Alabama. Some of the towns there do not even have names, but unfortunately some of the white locals know how to name and blame "the niggers" and "faggots" who were just getting what they deserved with this disease.[10] One young black woman, Sara, does not openly admit her diagnosis to anyone in her town but people suspect it because she looks ill.[11] Consequently, some of her neighbors stop bringing their children to play with Sara's own and people move out of the checkout line she stands in at the grocery store. Sara's silence about her AIDS was an attempted safeguard against being treated like someone with the plague, but it failed.

Silence about homosexuality or bisexuality within the black community is also an attempted safeguard against being treated like a social outcast and especially like a plague victim when AIDS is present. The black community has not been any more or less accepting of homosexuality as a sexual orientation than the white community has been. Giovanni Koll and Jaime Gutierrez explain the discrimination that accompanies homosexuality and feeds HIV stigma while also specifically addressing views of homosexuality within the black community. It is seen "as an embarrassment to the African American race" because it violates "gender roles and community norms about sexuality."[12] In his self-revealing and somewhat controversial *On the Down Low*, J.L. King explains that "when a man is called a fag, it hurts. It basically strips away your manhood."[13] This embarrassment about being gay or even bisexual within the black community can lead to "down low" behavior. These men cannot admit their sexuality to the women they are involved with, to their families, or to other social institutions, especially the church.

The stigma of homosexuality within the black community really stems from the same homophobia that pervades other communities, especially conservative whites who denigrated instead of helped the thousands of gay men perishing from AIDS in the early 1980s. Al Sharpton, a perennial activist against injustices affecting the African American community, explains that black homophobia is fed by whites because "blacks always want to be accepted by the white world, and the white world is homophobic."[14] Cathy Cohen views black homophobia as an "attempt" by black elites "to distance the community from blame and stigma."[15] By adopting a homophobic stance, blacks can join whites in a common effort to keep gays as *others* regardless of skin color.

Not surprisingly, gay and bisexual black men confronting an AIDS diagnosis tend to "hide their orientation," as Scott Jaschik puts it in an article that reviews a study of HIV incidence in the North Carolina male college population from 2000 to 2003. Eighty-four male students were found to have HIV and 73 of them were black. These black students presumably contracted the virus through sex with other men, but they did not feel comfortable enough admitting this, especially the men who also had sex with women.[16]

Sharpton offers a reason for this secretive activity in relation to the societal blame of AIDS victims. He calls on the black community, in particular church leaders, to stop asking "how" people contract the disease because the question inevitably leads to blame for getting it.[17] Or as I have phrased it, the societal focus on *who* gets the disease, especially gays and drug users, leads to offering them as human causes who then become scapegoats in the process of plague-making. Sharpton sees a connection between the blame bestowed upon people for contracting AIDS and the anticipated blame from society for just being gay or bisexual. The fear of blame consequently results in "down low" behavior. Men are on "the down low," he explains, "because they were pushed down low."[18] They were pushed down into hiding their sexuality by a society that is homophobic and by a society that has blamed homosexuals for the disease.

In addition, if AIDS was not persistently viewed and presented as a highly contagious disease that gay men were the original cause of, maybe not as many gay and bisexual black men would be so secretive about their sexuality. This homophobia, really gay hatred, within the black community and America at large has not fostered an environment of openness. And the plague-making of AIDS dropped another blanket over vocalization. Who wants to be ostracized for being gay and a plague carrier?

The silence produced by the interlaced stigma of being gay and having AIDS within the black community is captured by Cathy Cohen in her portrait of Billy. This young man cannot bring himself to reveal his HIV status to his working-class parents because "that would mean telling them that he was gay."[19] Billy seriously thought about an alternative. He could tell them that he shot drugs because that would be more acceptable to his family. King also captured this forced silence about homosexuality and AIDS when he describes the elaborate lie he and his good friend created in order to exonerate his friend from total alienation. King's friend is married and contracted AIDS through "down low" behavior. They decided this man would tell his wife that he had an indiscretion with a prostitute while out of town on business and unfortunately picked up the virus. Subsequently, he was able to hold on to his wife and the rest of his life by hiding his sexual orientation. King explains that "the black community could accept that this brother got the virus from a woman—even a prostitute. They could never accept that he got it from a man."[20]

For others in the black community, the very revelation of an AIDS diagnosis regardless of *how* it was contracted causes shame resulting in silence. King discusses the college-bound Nigel whose future was shattered, along with his girlfriend's, by AIDS. Nigel's unprotected rendezvous with a male photographer resulted in him contracting the virus, and he unwittingly in turn passed it on to his girlfriend. Nigel eventually died from AIDS but even his most intimate friends and family did not know what caused his death because his mother "did not want anybody to know he died from AIDS."[21] The cause of death on his death certificate was pneumonia, not AIDS. Even decades after AIDS emerged in America, Nigel's mother could not face her community if they knew her son died from the plague.

There is a "stifling stigma and silence" surrounding AIDS among southern blacks, according to Phill Wilson, who has been living with HIV for more than 20 years, that might explain Nigel's mother's response to AIDS if we can grant the Washington, D.C., area where he died southern status.[22] This stigma and silence have certainly affected the black community in Virginia where I have lived for the past four years. In early 2008, I attended a panel discussion at a college that was sponsored by a community AIDS taskforce. All of the male and female panelists worked for this organization; all of them were gay, black, and Virginia-born. All of them discussed their long journeys toward being accepted by their families, friends, and communities for being gay. All of them were practicing Christians and no one ever indicated a conflict between their religion and their sexuality, which I found curious. Most Baptist and Pentecostal preachers view homosexuality as a sin or at least as a perversion of morality. One of the panelists even talked about how she arrived at the acceptance that she was a sinner because she was gay!

I was disappointed that none of these men or women questioned the role of their religion in the discrimination they had faced their whole lives for being gay. As an outsider to Southern Christian African American culture, it was perhaps easier for me to see the role that religion played in their silence about being gay most of their lives. And that helped me to understand why, not even once, any of these panelists mentioned AIDS.

African American women share a reaction of silence to AIDS with the men in their community. This is indeed a sad reaction considering that by 2007 AIDS was "the top killer of black women 25 to 34 years old."[23] But the stigma surrounding AIDS produces a silence that allows many of the victims to escape discrimination and ostracism. During this time in Virginia, some women with HIV even refused to take their antiretroviral medication so that their respective boyfriends did not discover their diagnosis. This behavioral silence results in the virus itself growing out of control in these women's bodies and potentially leads to opportunistic infections resulting in a shortened life span. This powerful desire to hide their diagnosis in order to avoid isolation also leads to the potential spread of the virus to their sexual partners. These women probably did not request safer sex practices with their partners because that very request would raise the red flag they were trying to avoid. Many carriers of AIDS choose to be silent about their diagnosis because they do not want to experience the judgment that plague victims experience. This silence in turn can result in even more AIDS cases.

Artistic works also confirm this prevalent response to AIDS in the black community. The HBO movie *Life Support,* starring Queen Latifah as Anna, focuses on women with AIDS in New York City during the first decade of the twenty-first century. Anna helps run a support group for women with HIV. Anna and her husband, Slick, are HIV positive and we learn that they both converted around the same time back in their drug-using days. Both of them are open and honest about their HIV, unlike most of the women Anna supports in the group. We watch Anna, for instance, take her ARVs in front of her husband and Slick even prepares protein drinks for her. On the other hand, several women in the support group admit that they have a hard time telling new men in their lives that they are positive. One woman is terrified to tell her husband, and later we learn that she was killed, presumably by her husband after the revelation.[24]

Terry, who I cared for during the summer of 2006 in Baltimore, was not murdered by her husband for having HIV, but she felt forced into silence with former colleagues and even her own family. Terry was willing to wait two weeks for a blood transfusion in our outpatient center rather than immediately receiving one in the hospital where she used to work. Terry was a 37-year-old black female who contracted HIV in 1992. She had worked as a secretary on a surgical unit at the hospital where she would not go to get treated. Recently her CD4 count dropped precipitously low and placed her at great risk for infections and she had to quit work. Her antiretroviral drugs were subsequently intensified, which resulted in more toxic effects to her bone marrow—the reason she needed a blood transfusion.

Terry was petite, soft-spoken, and looked healthy. She attended some college years ago and proudly told me she had a 19-year-old daughter in college in Pennsylvania. She also had a 14-year-old boy. I apologized for the wait to get into our center for treatment and then asked her why she did not go to the hospital where she used to work, especially since her fatigue had worsened over the past two weeks and the blood would have alleviated it. "I used to work the 3–11 shift there and didn't want anyone to know my business," she revealed. "You mean, the AIDS?" I asked. She shook her head yes. She had worked there for years and no one knew she had AIDS and she did not feel comfortable enough to tell anyone. "Do you really think," I pressed, "if they found out now that they would treat you differently?" She was not so soft-spoken now. "Most definitely," she replied. It turns out that she did not even feel comfortable enough to tell her two children that she had AIDS. The two fathers of her children had disappeared years ago. She was not intimate with anyone at the time. I wondered if her son had even been tested for HIV because he was born the year she contracted it. I did not feel, however, that she wanted to pursue that line of speculation.

If Terry had cancer she could have comfortably returned as a patient to the hospital where she once worked for years. If any of her former colleagues had asked her why she needed a blood transfusion, she could have openly said, "I have cancer." Instead she avoided that place so she did not have to talk about having AIDS. If she had cancer, she would have felt comfortable enough explaining to her children why she had to quit work and take so many medications. Instead she suffered in silence with her stigmatizing disease within the most intimate world of her family.

The African American community is certainly not alone in responding to AIDS with reticence instead of vocalness. Interviews conducted by Robert Klitzman and Ronald Bayer of people living with HIV after the advent of the HAART era reveal that different ethnic, social, and sexual groups did not feel comfortable, privately or publically, revealing their HIV positive status. These two scientists interviewed more than 70 people: Some of them were white, some gay, some heterosexual, some poor, and some drug users. Although the interviewees were drawn from different groups, all of them overwhelmingly kept their HIV status a "secret from children, family members, and even healthcare providers."[25] The authors seemed surprised that in an era in which medications were now available to stop the once inevitable march to the grave from HIV, it was still so difficult for people to reveal their viral status. Yet, we have seen this difficulty time and time again since 1995.

A male Latino, former drug user struggled with telling his own girlfriend about his HIV. He felt like the right time never arrived. The interviewers interpreted his indecisiveness as stemming from "fears of rejection."[26] Other interviewees expressed this same fear when it came to the workplace and chose not to divulge their viral status in spite of antidiscrimination laws protecting people with disabilities that were in place during this time. One gay man who lived in a shelter and worked odd jobs felt that a disclosure would result in termination. Albeit he did not think it would be a blatant firing, rather it would be cloaked in other explanations, such as "oh, we ain't going to terminate you but we ain't got nothing for you to do."[27] Others felt fearful to reveal their diagnosis because it could result in the loss of a regular paycheck, as well as the insurance that helped to pay for the ARVs that kept them alive.

Even some health-care professionals with HIV chose silence over revelation in the workplace. This is not surprising, especially after so many of them witnessed the discrimination experienced by patients with AIDS and the hysteria generated around the Kimberly Bergalis case when she accused her dentist of giving her HIV during a procedure in the late 1980s.[28] The suspicion directed toward this dentist was enough for many patients to look at their own health-care providers with a discerning eye when it came to HIV transmission. One medical resident in the mid-1990s decided to remain silent about his HIV status in order to avoid judgment from colleagues and patients.[29] Even HIV positive nurses in 2006, in spite of having a voice through the Association of Nurses in AIDS Care's new committee for HIV positive nurses, felt like a divulgence of their positive status could place "their careers in jeopardy and they feared persecution by their medical colleagues."[30] Across ethnic, social, sexual, and professional groups, people living with HIV choose "silence not only to prevent isolation but to avoid being treated as different."[31] And people are treated differently because this disease has been viewed as a plague.

By 2006, 1 million people had HIV in the United States and a half of a million of them were dead from it.[32] In a population of almost 300 million AIDS affected about 3 percent of it, yet we still witness this disease being described as a plague. We have not lost half of the American population like the Europeans did in the fourteenth century from bubonic plague. One journalist declared in a 2001 article that "the most profound and immediate threat to life on earth is the AIDS epidemic," which he also calls a "plague."[33]

According to the CDC, a little more than 700,000 people were living with AIDS in the United States at this time—hardly the most "immediate threat" to human existence.[34] Poverty in our country constitutes a more immediate threat with 11.3 percent of the population enduring it when this article was written in 2001.[35] Poverty prevents not only adequate health care but disease prevention and consequently results in premature death from many otherwise controllable diseases, such as heart disease, diabetes, and HIV.

Plague-making hysteria continues to abound as the new century arrived. Bob Herbert reviews the history of AIDS in a 2001 article and begins by calling the disease not just *a* scourge but "*the* scourge."[36] Although his intentions are noble in discussing AIDS as a devastating disease that the United States responded too slowly to when it emerged and still does 20 years later, his hyperbolic statements about the global state of AIDS create panic about AIDS more than inspiration for a quicker response. Herbert sees that globally we are not prepared to battle AIDS that has taken over 20 million lives and "will soon surpass the lethal toll of the bubonic plague of the Middle Ages."[37] The global population in 2001 reached 6.1 billion and less than 1 percent of the world's population was dead from AIDS.[38] Herbert neglected to give his readers this global population statistic so that they could more rationally understand the actual percentage of people who have died. The more than 20 million people dead from AIDS seem earth-shattering when it stands alone.

Furthermore, contextualizing the number of AIDS deaths within the medieval bubonic plague diverts our attention away from the fact that AIDS has come nowhere near the death toll of 50–60 percent of a continent's population. Herbert secures AIDS position in the global plague narrative that began so long ago. And this position does nothing for encouraging people with AIDS to openly discuss their disease because it is still viewed as highly contagious and deadly.

Susan Hunter's call for the U.S. government—especially when George W. Bush and the Christian Right ruled the land—to respond more openly to AIDS by not restricting funds for prevention programs advocating safer sex, in part, drives her book *AIDS in America*. But this book also contributes to the hysteria that has surrounded the creation of AIDS as a plague as it bravely takes on the failures of our government in stemming this epidemic. In her introduction Hunter matter-of-factly refers to the disease as a plague when she asks, "Where are the voices of responsible leadership needed to counter this plague?"[39] Later she looks at the consequences of the U.S. government not acting quickly enough to halt the spread of this plague, and she imbibes the reader with a frightening fantasy regarding a magical new mode of transmission for HIV. The longer HIV is around, she argues, the more chance it has to mutate. Fair enough, and it has. But then, "imagine, for a moment, if AIDS became a respiratory infection and could be transmitted by a sneeze like the bubonic plague did when it became the Black Death in 1347."[40]

Pneumonic, *not* bubonic, plague could be transmitted by a sneeze because this form of *Yersinia pestis* infection infected lung tissue and could be found in the sputum. But pneumonic disease is different than bubonic even though each is caused by the same bacterium. Secondly, bubonic plague did not "become" the Black Death in 1347. The *Black Death* is a synonym for what we have traditionally viewed as the fourteenth-century plague and it was not coined until two centuries after this wave of bubonic disease. Facts about past plagues are distorted here as AIDS is "imagined" to be a highly contagious one. This type of plague-making perpetuates irrational responses to the illness, such as people not eating cookies baked by a 73-year-old woman with AIDS even in 2006.[41] It also explains why 51 percent of the American public in 2009, according to one poll, did not want their food prepared by someone with HIV.[42]

Some people, privately and publically, continued to think that the victims of AIDS deserved what they got because of certain behaviors. Offering human causes for this disease continues to be an intricate component in making it a plague, as Hunter shows us in some of the interviews she conducted with several Americans living with HIV. Many of these people do not fall into the traditional so-called risk groups for HIV. For example, Paige is a white, middle-class heterosexual from Montana who was in the process of being inducted into the Navy when her HIV test returned as positive. Paige's mother and sister are supportive as she struggles with the news but her stepfather feels differently.[43]

Apparently, Paige's stepfather had always been just a little bit disgusted with Paige's fast lifestyle in the past. When Paige's mother tells him about her diagnosis his response is judgmental. "She brought this all on herself," he says.[44] To him, AIDS was the natural consequence of what he viewed as unacceptable behavior—really it is the punishment for it. It is not hard to imagine in this type of atmosphere that Paige's primary reaction to her new diagnosis was feeling "dirty and shameful."[45] Paige's stepfather joins many other judges in determining who are "innocent" and "guilty" carriers of the virus.

More public judges of behavior continue to make their appearances in the first decade of this century. The Pat Buchanans and Jerry Falwells have not left the stage. President Bush nominated Jerry Thacker to the Presidential Advisory Council on HIV as 2002 turned into 2003 but this conservative Christian nominee, who became HIV positive in 1986 along with his wife and daughter secondary to a blood transfusion his wife received in 1984, was persuaded by the Department of Health and Human Services to withdraw his consideration for the position. Thacker called AIDS "the gay plague" and posted his biography on a Christian AIDS ministry website that further revealed his less- than-Christian approach to the disease.[46] He said that "AIDS was something that bad people had to worry about. Not Christians. Not the church."[47] Thacker certainly did not consider that he and his own family must qualify as these "bad people" since they had to worry about AIDS. He withdrew as a candidate from the presidential council.

A state official in Maryland, Comptroller William Donald Schaefer, publically stated in October 2004 that people with AIDS were "a danger" and "brought it on themselves."[48] These statements perpetuate the view that AIDS is a plague—a highly contagious disease whose victims deserve it. Schaefer actually said this in order to clarify earlier statements regarding how Maryland should create a public registry listing the names of all people who are HIV positive. Early in the epidemic, AIDS activists fought against this exact list because people even suspected of having the disease lost their jobs, promotions, and medical insurance. More than two decades after the epidemic emerged in the United States, people with HIV did not feel any more confident that such a registry would result in anything other than the discrimination wielded by this public official who proposed it.

Furthermore, people with HIV also fear criminal conviction for carrying the virus, especially since 27 states made HIV transmission a felony by 2000.[49] The perceived plague carrier has been criminalized like the Jews who were accused of spreading bubonic plague in early fourteenth-century Europe. Of course the Jews were executed for their supposed offense, whereas people with the modern plague faced more minor legal punishments.

The cultural persistence in creating this disease as a plague along with proposals to publically reveal carriers and potentially turn them into criminals leaves the person with HIV little choice but to remain silent. The case of a woman recently convicted of prostitution and potentially transmitting HIV to an undercover police officer in the Virginia Beach region epitomizes our lack of progress as a society in viewing AIDS more rationally and less like a plague. This 45-year-old woman agreed to have sexual intercourse with two police officers in exchange for money in June 2010. The case also involved determining whether or not she was guilty of "infected sexual battery" because she was HIV positive. The one officer testified that before the sale of sex was offered by the defendant, he asked her "if she was clean" and she answered affirmatively.[50] Of course this question really means, "Do you have AIDS?" These officers knew she had AIDS from her previous conviction of prostitution one year earlier. Having HIV is synonymous with being dirty and sinful while being negative means one is clean and pure, or untarnished by the plague. This woman is made to be the responsible one for transmission of HIV because she is the perceived plague vector. How do we know that the officer is not carrying the virus? The focus remains on the *who* instead of on the *how* of transmission.

The judge in this case was skeptical that this convicted prostitute intended to infect the officers who entrapped her because her crack addiction was viewed as skewing her judgment in revealing her viral status to potential clients. Yet she was convicted of the lesser misdemeanor of "failing to disclose her HIV status to an intended sexual partner."[51] If she did admit her HIV positive status, she ran the risk of being convicted of infected sexual battery. Reticence will continue to dominate the reaction spectrum of the HIV carrier until the disease becomes destigmatized, or deplagued.

Conclusions: The Legacy of Plague-Making

In spite of the stigma that surrounds AIDS and the discrimination that has been endured by most people carrying the virus, amazing medical advances have been made in treating this disease. By 2010, there were approximately 30 FDA-approved antiretroviral medications to treat HIV infection.[1] Many of these are combination drugs that facilitate compliance in taking a large number of pills and in turn increase survival rates. Before these antiretrovirals, the median survival of a person with AIDS was one and a half years, but today the median survival has increased to 14.9 years.[2]

New drugs in clinical trials bind to receptors on white blood cells, which HIV uses to enter the cells, and halt the very process of infection. More traditional antiretrovirals that induce cell destruction after the virus has already invaded the cell continue to be developed, as well. In other trials, chemotherapy drugs used to treat cancer of the lung and pancreas and even leukemia are demonstrating destructive action against HIV.

The medical field also has been moving toward routine screening for HIV disease, like we perform for cholesterol levels. In 2003, with the recognition that the number of new HIV cases in the United States remained at a steady 40,000 per annum, the CDC created the Advancing HIV Prevention initiative for preventing HIV. Its major focus was to require every American between 13 and 64 to get tested at least once.[3] At least if people knew their HIV status baseline, they could appropriately practice safer sex—so this logic goes. Those people at high risk are recommended for testing annually. Remnants of the classic risk groups, unfortunately, still linger as the CDC defines high risk, in part, as "injection drug users, persons who exchange sex for money and drugs, and men who have sex with men."[4] At least "homosexuals" are removed from the list, and the CDC attempts parity in this high-risk definition by including heterosexuals "who themselves or whose sex partner have had more than one sex partner" since their most recent test.[5] I would have liked to see this high-risk list simply defined as anyone who engages in sexual behavior that is unprotected or shares any drug instruments, instead of the persistent categorizing of marginal groups in our society as "high risk" because the disease will remain affiliated with them alone.

Nonetheless, the CDC's goal in implementing routine testing is to "reduce the stigma as well as transmission" of HIV. If an HIV test is "as common as a cholesterol check,"[6] as this agency wants, and if everyone is tested initially regardless of their risk, then we as a society should move away from treating the disease like a plague. But the implementation of this testing has been slow, to say the least. I have not witnessed routine testing as a nurse in any setting, and I have never been offered it by any of my own doctors.

Until HIV testing becomes routine for everyone, we will continue to think that the disease only happens to certain groups of people who deserve to get it because of what they have done. And until we stop blaming people for the disease, it will continue to be viewed as a plague. Patient Zero hunting was still happening, for example, in early 2005 when AIDS scientists thought a "super virus" emerged because one man in New York City developed full-blown AIDS only months after he tested negative for the virus, and the virus he had was already resistant to many antiretroviral drugs. Instead of focusing on the highly drug-resistant strain of HIV this man acquired, one journalist focused on his sexual orientation, including details of his sex life. He was "gay" and "had more than 100 sexual contacts over the past six months." In addition, his sexual activities were "unprotected while under the influence of methamphetamine."[7] He is another Patient Zero in the AIDS plague narrative that had been initiated in 1981 when the first group of sex-and-drug crazed gay men with KS was presented as such by the CDC and other journalists.

This journalist also talks about how the health department was desperately searching for this man's sexual partners, presumably to warn them of their contact with this new Patient Zero who carries the supervirus. But alas, one of his sexual partners had been infected with HIV for years. The Patient Zero theory collapsed. Again we are reminded that one person cannot be held responsible for spreading HIV regardless of the strain. Again we are reminded that any type of Patient Zero theory is a convenient excuse to find a human scapegoat for this human-made plague. It is indeed amazing that gay men instead of the virus itself once again are still presented as the cause of AIDS.

Until we stop calling AIDS a plague, people will not feel comfortable rationally discussing it. As recent as the spring of 2010, a journalist covering the closing of St. Vincent's Hospital in New York City described one nurse's experience there with "the mystifying and terrifying AIDS plague of the 1980s and 1990s."[8] We need to demystify the illness so that when gay people without AIDS deal with a cancer diagnosis, for example, they do not fear judgment for having AIDS. In her article on gay patients with cancer, Anne Katz describes one gay man's fear regarding assumptions about his weight loss after cancer surgery. He says, "I wondered if it was going to be perceived within the gay community as having AIDS."[9] Almost three decades after the emergence of AIDS in the United States, this man feels like a cancer diagnosis is more acceptable than an AIDS one.

My own brother-in-law felt the same way when doctors were trying to diagnose the ultimate origin of his sudden onset of pericarditis (an inflammation of the sac around the heart) in 2007. Joe visited the hospital so often that summer that the family began to view it as his vacation home. But August 5 was different. The doctors were buzzing about pericardial mesothelioma— a type of cancer that invades the sac around the heart. A death sentence indeed. Chemotherapy is ineffective at best. Surgery and radiation are not even options. The time from diagnosis to the end is approximately two months. My sister called to ask me to talk with Joe because the infectious disease doctors wanted to test him for HIV in order to rule out a viral type of pericarditis (CMV) seen in some people with AIDS. Unlike mesothelioma, this disease would be treatable. The problem was that Joe did not want to consent to the HIV test. He told me, "I never screwed a guy and I never shot drugs." And then, "What will people think?" There's that old refrain spoken by people who do not want to face the discrimination that has been AIDS' companion for so long in American society.

My brother-in-law was facing a fatal cancer diagnosis and he seemed more terrified of a potential AIDS one. The plague-making of AIDS had been so successful that in the absolute hour of his desperation, dying from cancer seemed more palatable than living with AIDS. He consented to the test, which revealed no HIV. The cancer was never confirmed, either. I asked him recently if I could include his experience here because it illustrates how the plague-making of AIDS has permeated the American psyche.

And yet, I thought, or perhaps romantically hoped, that when I returned to caring for AIDS patients on a daily basis on an oncology unit once again in 2010, the effects of this plague-making had evaporated. I met Joy when a new nurse asked me to start her IV for the chemotherapy she was about to receive for her newly diagnosed Burkitt's lymphoma. I had not seen that diagnosis in a long time. This type of lymphoma invades the abdomen and it is one of the cancers that patients with AIDS can get. Joy was diagnosed with HIV in 1991 and never had any opportunistic infections or cancer until now—I learned this when I was alone in her room later that week. We had a lot in common. It turned out that she had lived in New York City when I did. She lost a friend to AIDS every month and I lost a patient every night. We wore different robes through the worst years of the epidemic. I reminded her how lucky she was to be alive. She knew. The lilies were in her room also. Maybe I could finally alter my response to them.

On the first of May, I was not convinced that I could smell those lilies and not think of Larry and his death when I received report from the night nurse. Joy had never recovered from her last round of chemotherapy almost three weeks ago. She was not her perky self—chatting with friends, making business deals over the phone, and eating her favorite gourmet take-out food. "She might have KS in her lungs," the night nurse told me. My heart sank. Larry was not too far away. Those lilies emitted their painful scent.

Joy asked to see me and she wanted to know more about her potential diagnosis. The bronchoscopy results that would reveal the cancer were not finalized. The pulmonologist's initial report said, "it could be KS." I needed to stick to the facts as I answered her questions. There was no KS diagnosis yet and there might not be. And I needed to leave Larry at the door as I entered her room.

Joy and I got to know each other pretty well over the past few months. She trusted my knowledge of AIDS and cancer and my honesty. She asked me what it would mean if she did have KS in her lungs. I explained that still there was no cure for it and her time would be shorter than longer. She looked up at me from the pictures she had been shuffling in her hands. In between beautiful self-portraits were the bronchoscopy pictures of the faintly purplish lesions in her lungs.

When her two devoted friends, Tom and Dave, arrived that evening, Tom told me in the hallway that he had been talking to Joy about making her final arrangements, but she was resistant. He also revealed to me that only he, Dave, and Joy's mother knew her AIDS diagnosis. I thought the parade of daily visitors knew. I asked why only them. "We are the only ones left," Tom said. "Yes. Of course," I thought of Petrarch's letter to Boccaccio, "of all my friends, only you remain." And I was reminded once again in 2010 how much AIDS felt like a plague to this close-knit gay community. I asked Tom why none of Joy's visitors knew. Tom said, "I guess she didn't feel comfortable telling anyone else." I guess not. And then I remembered Joy telling me a few months ago during one of our stolen conversations in her room that she did not feel *quite* as ostracized for having AIDS now like she did when she was first diagnosed. Now when people, especially health-care workers, know her AIDS diagnosis, they are not blatantly critical, but "don't want to talk too much, touch too much, or spend too much time around you," she revealed. Guarded discrimination of the perceived plague carrier certainly persisted.

Joy has been living with AIDS for almost 20 years. The KS diagnosis was negative. The purplish lesions in her lungs were not KS, after all, but little bruises from her low platelet count produced by the intense chemotherapy she received. Joy's lungs indeed would heal. She had her last round of chemotherapy at the end of the summer. I hugged her and said good-bye since she would not need to be hospitalized for treatment again. I wished her luck in her next business venture. This was the first time I said good-bye to an AIDS patient who would go on living.

AIDS is not a plague. No disease is a plague. *Plague* is a cultural construct—a label usually applied to contagious diseases in which marginal groups of people in any given society are scapegoated by more socially powerful and acceptable ones. Yet many victims of the disease also see it as a plague in order to express the suffering of their own and their communities', such as American gays and blacks. From their perspective, AIDS swiftly killed so many of their own and the *plague* label captured this experience.

Calling a disease a plague, however, primarily facilitates continual blame to be bestowed upon certain people and behaviors while exonerating the socially acceptable from responsibility in dealing with the disease. If these "acceptables" happen to contract the disease that has been made a plague, they consider themselves innocent and maintain the mistaken understanding that the guilty (the "unacceptables") are responsible for it: the poor, the unorthodox, the Jew, the Chinese, the gay, and the drug user, to name a few. Plague-making has been a powerful centuries-long process of justifying discrimination epidemiologically.

If AIDS had not been created as a plague, especially a gay one originally, Americans might have sympathized, or at least not demonized, the disease's victims when it swiftly killed them. We even might have embraced them when the viral cause was discovered and when medications were found to defer death.

Of the many people with AIDS I have cared for over the past 25 years, I have never met one person who has not experienced discrimination on some level. As a country, as human beings, we should have done better in dealing with and contributing to the discrimination that has enveloped this epidemic. We could have done better. We can always begin by extending a gloveless hand and not letting go.

Notes

Chapter 1

1. "The New Plague, in Perspective," *The New York Times,* September 3, 1985, p. A20.
2. *Morbidity and Mortality Weekly Report,* June 5, 1981, 30(21): 250–2 and *MMWR,* July 3, 1981, 30(25): 305–8.
3. For AIDS statistics see Robin Marantz Henig, "AIDS: A New Disease's Deadly Odyssey," *The New York Times,* February 6, 1983, p. SM 28 and for "gay plague" see Dudley Clendinen, "AIDS Spreads Pain and Fear among Ill and Healthy Alike," *The New York Times,* June 17, 1983, p. A1.
4. Ole J. Benedictow, *The Black Death 1346–1353: The Complete History* (Woodbridge: The Boydell Press, 2004), p. 377.
5. See Michael B.A. Oldstone, *Viruses, Plagues, and History* (Oxford: Oxford University Press, 1998), p. 27 for small pox statistics and p. 30 for references to the disease as plague. See Gina Kolata, *Flu: The Story of the Great Influenza Pandemic of 1918 and the Search for the Virus that Caused It* (New York: Simon and Schuster, 1999), p. 7 for the 1918 influenza statistics and Chapter 1 for references to it as plague. See Richard L. Bruno, "Polio: The Sequel," *Advance for Nurses,* April 11, 2005: 15–17 for references to polio as plague.
6. Clendinen, "AIDS Spreads Pain and Fear."
7. Ibid.
8. For this statistic see Glenn Collins, "Facing the Emotional Anguish of AIDS," *The New York Times,* May 30, 1983, p. 14.
9. Clendinen, "AIDS Spreads Pain and Fear."
10. Benedictow, p. 213.
11. See Lawrence K. Altman, "Making Rounds: AIDS Rooms," *The New York Times,* January 3, 1984, p. C1. Altman is a medical doctor and observed that some of his colleagues and medical students "have become so frightened that they have refused to treat AIDS patients."
12. See "The New Plague, in Perspective," *The New York Times,* September 3, 1985, p. A20.

Chapter 2

1. *Morbidity and Mortality Weekly Report,* July 2, 1993; 42(25): 481–86.
2. Homer, *The Iliad,* trans. and ed. Richmond Lattimore (Chicago and London: The University of Chicago Press, 1951), bk 1, line 61.

3. *The Oxford English Dictionary*, 2d ed., s.v "plague."
4. Homer *Iliad* 1. 52.
5. Ibid., 1. 47–48.
6. Ibid., 1. 97.
7. Ibid., 1. 42
8. Thucydides, *History of the Peloponnesian War*, trans. Rex Warner (London: Penguin Books, 1954).
9. Thucydides 2.47.
10. See Michael B.A. Oldstone, *Viruses, Plagues, and History* (Oxford: Oxford University Press, 1998), chps. 4, 5, and 6 for a concise overview on the symptoms of smallpox, yellow fever, and measles.
11. Ibid., p. 33.
12. Ibid., p. 29.
13. Thucydides 2.50.
14. Ibid., 2.48.
15. Ibid., 1.22.
16. *The Holy Bible: A Translation from the Latin Vulgate in the Light of the Hebrew and Greek Originals*, trans. Ronald Knox (New York: Sheed and Ward, Inc, 1944), Gen 12:2. This modern English translation of Jerome's original Latin bible from 390–405 CE is invaluable because it makes available the version of the bible used by the medieval world, which is the focus of the next chapter. This version is used for all biblical references.
17. Gen. 12:17–18.
18. 1 Kings 5: 6–7.
19. See Jerome Goddard, "Fleas and Plague" *Infectious Medicine* 16, no. 1 (1999): 21–23 for bubonic plague symptoms, transmission, and the course of illness.
20. Apoc. 3:10.
21. Apoc. 21:27.
22. Apoc. 14:7.
23. Apoc. 14:6.
24. Apoc. 9:18.
25. Apoc. 9:20.
26. Apoc. 16:2.
27. Apoc. 15:1–2.
28. Apoc. 16:6–7.
29. Apoc. 16:18.
30. Apoc. 6:8.

Chapter 3

1. See *Morbidity and Mortality Weekly Report*, November 30, 1999, 39 (RR-16): 27–31.
2. See respectively Norman Cantor, *In the Wake of the Plague* (New York: The Free Press, 2001), p. 6 and Mark Wheelis, "Biological Warfare at the 1346 Siege of Caffa," *Emerging Infectious Disease* 8, no. 9 (2002), pp. 971–975.

3. Ole J. Benedictow, *The Black Death 1346–1353: The Complete History* (Woodbridge: The Boydell Press, 2004), pp. 382–383.
4. Robert S. Gottfried, *The Black Death: Natural and Human Disaster in Medieval Europe* (New York: The Free Press, 1983), p. 38.
5. Giovanni Boccaccio, *The Decameron*, trans. G.H. McWilliam (London: Penguin, 1972), p. 57.
6. Boccaccio, p. 58.
7. See Benedictow, p. 291.
8. Raymond Crawfurd, *Plague and Pestilence in Literature and Art* (Oxford: Clarendon Press, 1914), p. 111.
9. Benedictow, p. 276.
10. See Philip Ziegler, *The Black Death* (New York: Harper and Row Publishers, 1969), p. 79.
11. See *The Black Death*, ed. and trans. Rosemary Horrox (Manchester and New York: Manchester University Press, 1994), p. 77.
12. Horrox, p. 3.
13. Ibid., pp. 24–25.
14. Ibid., p. 74.
15. See "Imported Plague—New York City 2002," *MMWR*, August 20, 2003, 52(31): 725–728.
16. See "Human Plague—Four States, 2006," *MMWR*, September 1, 2006, 55 (44): 940–943.
17. See Gottfried, p. 26.
18. See Horrox, p. 7 and John Kelly, *The Great Mortality: An Intimate History of the Black Death, the Most Devastating Plague of All Time* (New York: Harper Perennial, 2005), p. 19.
19. Horrox, p. 83.
20. See Wheelis, "Biological Warfare."
21. Horrox, p. 17.
22. Benedictow, p. 91.
23. Horrox, p. 183.
24. Benedictow, p. 236.
25. Graham Twigg, *The Black Death: A Biological Reappraisal* (New York: Schocken Books, 1985), p. 111.
26. Ibid., p. 213.
27. See Brian Fagan, *The Little Ice Age* (New York: Basic Books, 2000).
28. Cantor, p. 15.
29. Benedictow, p. 22.
30. Kelly, pp. 113, 300.
31. Cantor, p. 16.
32. *The Middle English Dictionary*, s.v. "plàge."
33. Benedictow, p. 5.
34. Benedictow, p. 127.
35. William Langland, *The Vision of William Concerning Piers the Plowman Together with Vita de Dowel, Dobet, et Dobest*, ed. W.W. Skeat, The Early English Text

Society (London: Oxford University Press, 1869). This edition of the poem is in the original Middle English and I translate the lines cited.

36. Langland, Passus V, line 13.
37. Geoffrey Chaucer, *The Canterbury Tales*, in *The Riverside Chaucer*, third edition, general ed. Larry D. Benson (Boston: Houghton Mifflin Company, 1987). I translate the lines of Chaucer's Middle English into modern English.
38. Chaucer, "The Wife of Bath's Tale," line 1264.
39. Chaucer, "The Pardoner's Tale," line 679.
40. Horrox, p. 59.
41. Ibid., p. 58.
42. Boccaccio, pp. 49, 51, 54.
43. *The Middle English Dictionary,* s.v. "scourge."
44. The June 28, 2007 democratic presidential debate was live from Howard University in Washington D.C. and aired on UNC PBS channel 6 in Norfolk, VA.
45. Horrox, pp. 159–161.
46. Ibid., p. 59.
47. Chaucer, "The Knight's Tale," line 2469.
48. Boccaccio, p. 50.
49. Horrox, p. 15.
50. Ibid., p. 126. This poem is in prose form.
51. Ibid., p. 134.
52. Ibid., p. 11.
53. Ziegler, pp. 81–82.
54. Horrox, p. 134.
55. Ibid., pp. 117, 118.
56. Langland, Passus X, lines 75, 77.
57. Horrox, p. 133.
58. Ibid., pp 15–16.
59. Chaucer, "General Prologue," cf. lines 165–207.
60. Horrox, p. 75.
61. Ibid., p. 246.
62. Francesco Petrarch, "The Triumph of Death," trans. Mary Sidney Herbert, in *Petrarch in English*, ed. Thomas P. Roche, Jr. (London: Penguin Books, 2005), line 145. I modernized the spelling of this line.
63. See "Sonnet 310" in *Petrarch: Selections from the Canzoniere and Other Works*, ed. and trans. Mark Musa (Oxford: Oxford University Press, 1985), p. 68.
64. Gottfried, p. 93.
65. See Norman Davies, *Europe: A History. A Panorama of Europe, East and West, from the Ice Age to the Cold War, from the Urals to Gibraltar* (New York: Harper Perennial, 1996), p. 411.
66. Chaucer, "The Book of the Duchess," line 11.
67. "The Book of the Duchess," lines 587–588.
68. Boccaccio, p. 52.

69. Horrox, p. 58.
70. Horrox, p. 61.
71. Benedictow, p. 214.
72. Cantor, p. 213.
73. Philippa Tristram, *Figures of Life and Death in Medieval English Literature* (New York: NYU Press, 1976), p. 15.
74. Raymond Crawfurd, *Plague and Pestilence in Literature and Art* (Oxford: Clarendon Press, 1914), p. 134.
75. Boccaccio, p. 52.
76. Ziegler, p. 71.
77. Boccaccio, p. 54.
78. Gottfried, p. 52.
79. John Mandeville, *The Travels of Sir John Mandeville*, trans. C.W.R.D. Moseley (London and New York: Penguin Books, 1983), p. 105.
80. Ibid., p. 132.
81. Crawfurd, p. 43.
82. Ibid., p. 48.
83. Horrox, p. 109.
84. Ibid., p. 212.
85. See Ziegler, p. 101.
86. Horrox, p. 219.
87. See Davies, p. 412.
88. Horrox, p. 221.
89. Ibid., p. 221.
90. Ibid., p. 208.
91. Ibid.
92. Ibid., p. 210.
93. Ibid., p. 219.
94. Ibid., p. 220.
95. See Davies, p. 412.
96. Horrox, p. 207.

Chapter 4

1. See Robert S. Gottfried, *The Black Death: Natural and Human Disaster in Medieval Europe* (New York: The Free Press, 1983), pp. 130–133. He discusses these plague recurrences throughout Europe after the mid-fourteenth century one.
2. John Lydgate, "A Dietary, and a Doctrine for Pestilence," in *The Minor Poems of John Lydgate*, ed. Henry Noble MacCracken, The Early English Text Society (London: Oxford University Press, 1934), lines 2, 5, 8, 16, and 24. I translate all lines from this poem into modern English.
3. Ibid., line 152.

4. See Philippa Tristam, *Figures of Life and Death in Medieval English Literature* (New York: New York University Press, 1976), plate 25.
5. See Carol Rawcliffe, *Medicine and Society in Later Medieval England* (London: Sutton Publishing Limited, 1995), plate 15.
6. See Tristam, pp. 160–161.
7. This painting was completed circa 1562 and resides in *The Prada* in Madrid, Spain. I have a reprint of it in my home.
8. Raymond Crawfurd, *Plague and Pestilence in Literature and Art* (Oxford: Clarendon Press, 1914), pp. 157–158.
9. Ibid., p. 158.
10. Barbara Howard Traister, *The Notorious Astrological Physician of London: Works and Days of Simon Forman* (Chicago and London: The University of Chicago Press, 2001), pp. 44–47.
11. Ibid., p. 45.
12. Ibid.
13. Ibid., p. 46.
14. A. Lloyd Moote and Dorothy C. Moote, *The Great Plague: The Story of London's Most Deadly Year* (Baltimore and London: The Johns Hopkins University Press, 2004), p. 19.
15. Ibid. pp. 10–11, 250.
16. Samuel Pepys, *The Diary of Samuel Pepys: A Selection*, ed. Robert Lantham (London and New York: Penguin Books, 1985).
17. John Dryden "Annus Mirabilis, The Year of Wonders, 1666," in *Selected Poetry and Prose of John Dryden,* ed. Earl Miner (New York: The Modern Library, 1969).
18. Daniel Defoe, *A Journal of the Plague Year,* ed. Cynthia Wall (London and New York: Penguin Books, 2003).
19. Pepys, May 24, 1665, p. 491.
20. Defoe, pp. 100, 74.
21. Defoe's original title is reprinted in Cynthia Wall's edition.
22. Defoe, p. 17.
23. Moote and Moote, p. 67.
24. Pepys, October 16, 1665, pp. 543–544.
25. Moote and Moote, p. 21.
26. Dryden, stanza 266.
27. Ibid., lines 1162–63.
28. Defoe, p. 21.
29. See Moote and Moote, p. 70.
30. Pepys, December 22, 1665, p. 563.
31. See Graham Twigg, *The Black Death: A Biological Reappraisal* (New York: Schocken Books, 1985), p. 117.
32. Moote and Moote, p. 71.
33. Defoe, p. 12.
34. Ibid., p. 13.
35. Ibid., p. 73.

36. See Defoe, Appendix I, p. 243.
37. See Moote and Moote, pp. 70–71.
38. Pepys, June 17, 1665, p. 498 and July 29, 1665, p. 509.
39. Defoe, p. 184.
40. Ibid., p. 195.
41. Pepys, July 29, 1666, p. 647.
42. Defoe, p. 234.
43. Moote and Moote, p. 178.
44. Pepys, September 30, 1665, p. 536.
45. Moote and Moote, pp. 79, 89.
46. Defoe, p. 190.
47. Pepys, October 7, 1665, p. 539.
48. Defoe, p. 116.
49. Moote and Moote, pp. 205–206.
50. See Defoe, pp. 63–65.
51. See Moote and Moote, p. 55.
52. Ibid., pp. 115–116.
53. See Defoe, p. 76.
54. See Pepys, September 3, 1665, p. 520.
55. See Gottfried, p. 52; Crawfurd, p. 162, and Defoe, p. 37.
56. See Moote and Moote, p. 53.
57. Pepys, June 7, 1665, p. 494.
58. See Defoe, p. 29.
59. Ibid., p. 153.
60. Ibid., pp. 68–69.
61. Moote and Moote, p. 81.
62. Ibid., p. 66.
63. See Defoe, p. 81.
64. Moote and Moote, p. 194.
65. Ibid., p. 47.
66. *The Oxford English Dictionary*, 2d ed., s.v "sluttish."

Chapter 5

1. See Ole J. Benedictow, *The Black Death 1346–1353: The Complete History* (Woodbridge: The Boydell Press, 2004), p. XV.
2. Myron Echenberg, *Plague Ports: The Global Urban Impact of Bubonic Plague: 1894–1901* (New York and London: New York University Press, 2007), p. xi.
3. Ibid., p. 17.
4. Edward Marriott, *Plague: A Story of Science, Rivalry, and the Scourge that Won't Go Away* (New York: Henry Holt and Company, 2002), p. 25.
5. Echenberg, p. 15.
6. Ibid., Appendix, p. 314.
7. Ibid.

8. Marriott, p. 61 and Echenberg, p. 27.
9. Marriott, p. 93.
10. Ibid., p. 30.
11. Echenberg, p. 35.
12. Marriott, p. 147.
13. John Kelly, *The Great Mortality: An Intimate History of the Black Death, the Most Devastating Plague of All Time* (New York: Harper Perennial, 2005), p. 41
14. Marriott, p. 61.
15. Ibid., p. 55.
16. Ibid., pp. 59–60.
17. Marilyn Chase, *The Barbary Plague: The Black Death in Victorian San Francisco* (New York: Random House Trade Paperbacks, 2003), pp. 12–13.
18. Ibid., p. 71.
19. Ibid., p. 5.
20. Ibid., pp. 4, 48.
21. Ibid., p. 12.
22. Echenberg, p. 224.
23. Chase, p. 11.
24. Ibid., p. 46.
25. Ibid., p. 168.
26. Ibid., p. 163.
27. Ibid., p. 179.
28. Marriott, pp. 230–231 and James Cross Giblin, *When Plague Strikes: The Black Death, Small Pox, AIDS* (New York: Harper Collins Publishers, 1995), p. 51.
29. Marriott, p. 180.
30. John F. Burns, "Thousands Flee Indian City in Deadly Plague Outbreak," *The New York Times,* September 24, 1994.
31. John F. Burns, "Plague Cases Confirmed in Region across India," *The New York Times,* September 28, 1994.
32. "Experts Call for Easing Plague Precautions on Travel from India," *The New York Times*, October 26, 1994.
33. Burns, "Thousands Flee Indian City in Deadly Plague Outbreak."
34. Ibid.
35. "Return of the Plague," *The New York Times,* September 29, 1994.
36. Ibid.
37. Herman Hesse, *Narcisus and Goldmund*, trans. Ursule Molinaro (New York: The Noonday Press, 1930), pp. 199–230.
38. Albert Camus, *The Plague*, trans. Stuart Gilbert (New York: Vintage International, 1948), pp. 6, 3.
39. Ibid., pp. 95, 98.
40. Ibid., p. 113.
41. Ibid., p. 181.
42. *Panic in the Streets*, dir. Elia Kazan, Twentieth Century Fox, 1950 and *The Seventh Seal*, dir. Ingmar Bergman, Criterion, 1957.

43. *The Seventh Seal.*
44. Benedictow, p. 171.
45. Kelly, p. 23.
46. *The Seventh Seal.*
47. Ibid.
48. Gina Kolata, *Flu: The Story of the Great Influenza Pandemic of 1918 and the Search for the Virus that Caused It* (New York: Simon and Schuster, 1999), pp. 5, 7.
49. John Barry, "Lessons from the 1918 Flu," *Time,* October 17, 2005, p. 96.
50. Kolata, pp. 3, 7.
51. Katherine Anne Porter, "Pale Horse, Pale Rider" in *The Collected Stories of Katherine Anne Porter* (San Diego: Harcourt, Brace and Company, 1944), pp. 269–317 and *The Holy Bible: A Translation from the Latin Vulgate in the Light of the Hebrew and Greek Originals,* trans. Ronald Knox (New York: Sheed and Ward, Inc, 1944), Apoc. 6:8.
52. Porter, pp. 281, 299.
53. Stephen King, *The Stand* (New York: Doubleday and Company, Inc., 1978).
54. King, p. 166.
55. Ibid., p. 24.

Chapter 6

1. *Morbidity and Mortality Weekly Report,* June 5, 1981, 30(21): 250–252.
2. Ibid., pp. 250, 251.
3. Ibid., p. 251.
4. *MMWR,* July 3, 1981, 30(25): 305–308.
5. Ibid., p. 305.
6. Ibid., p. 306.
7. Ibid.
8. Lawrence K. Altman, "Rare Cancer Seen in 41 Homosexuals," *The New York Times,* July 3, 1981.
9. Ibid.
10. Ibid.
11. Ibid.
12. Ibid.
13. See Martin Duberman, *Stonewall* (New York: Plume, 1993), pp. 97, 99.
14. See Larry Kramer, *The Destiny of Me* in *Two Plays: The Normal Heart and the Destiny of Me* (New York: Grove Press, 2000).
15. Duberman, p. 99.
16. Ibid., p. 201.
17. Ibid., p. 202.
18. R. L. Spitzer, "The Diagnostic Status of Homosexuality in DSM-III: A Reformulation of the Issues," *American Journal of Psychiatry,* 138 (1981): 210–215 discusses the removal of homosexuality as a mental disorder from the DSM-II and its addition as a "sexual orientation disturbance." In 1986,

homosexuality was completely removed from the manual. See also "Facts about Homosexuality and Mental Health" @ http://psychology.ucdavis.edu/rainbow/HTML/facts-mental-health.

19. Bruce Schulman, *The Seventies: The Great Shift in American Culture, Society, and Politics* (Cambridge, MA: Da Capo Press, 2001), p. 94.

20. Ibid., p. 96.

21. Ibid., p. 92.

22. Ibid., p. 41.

23. Ibid., p. 202.

24. Cindy Patton, "The New Right" in *While the World Sleeps: Writing from the First Twenty Years of the Global AIDS Plague*, ed. Chris Bull (New York: Thunder's Mouth Press, 2003), p. 40.

25. See Michael Gottlieb et al., "Pneumocystis carinii Pneumonia and Mucosal Candidiasis in Previously Healthy Homosexual Men," *New England Journal of Medicine* 305, no. 24 (December 10, 1981): 1425–1431.

26. Ibid., p. 1429.

27. Ibid., p. 1431.

28. "Two Fatal Diseases Focus of Inquiry: Rare Cancer and Pneumonia in Homosexual Men Studied," *The New York Times*, August 29, 1981.

29. Lawrence K. Altman, "New Homosexual Disorder Worries Health Officials," *The New York Times*, May 11, 1982.

30. "Two Fatal Diseases."

31. Altman, "New Homosexual Disorder."

32. Jean Seligmann et al., "The AIDS Epidemic: The Search for a Cure," *Newsweek*, April 18, 1983, p. 74.

33. Robin Marantz Henig, "AIDS: A New Disease's Deadly Odyssey," *The New York Times*, February 6, 1983, p. SM28.

34. Ibid.

35. Eileen Keerdoja and Holly Morris, "Homosexual Plague Strikes New Victims," *Newsweek*, August 23, 1982, p. 10.

36. Ibid.

37. For the number of AIDS cases see Robin Herman, "A Disease's Spread Provokes Anxiety," *The New York Times*, August 8, 1982, p. 31.

38. Seligmann, p. 74.

39. Keerdoja and Morris, p. 10.

40. Lawrence E. Lockman, *The AIDS Epidemic: A Citizen's Guide to Protecting Your Family and Community from the Gay Plague* (Ramona, California: Vic Lockman, 1986), p. 6.

41. Ibid., p. 8.

42. Ibid.

43. Larry Kramer, "1,112 and Counting" in *Reports from the Holocaust* (New York: St. Martin's Press, 1989), pp. 33–51.

44. Henig, "AIDS: A New Disease's Deadly Odyssey."

45. Kramer, "1,112," p. 33.

46. *An Early Frost*, dir. John Erman, NBC, November 11, 1985.
47. Ibid.
48. Henig, "AIDS: A New Disease's Deadly Odyssey."
49. Ibid.
50. Seligmann et al., "The AIDS Epidemic: The Search for a Cure."
51. Anne Gray, "A 20th century plague," *Nursing Times* 79, no. 35 (1983): 8–10.
52. Ibid.
53. Chris Bull, introduction to *While the World Sleeps*, p. xvii.
54. Kramer, "2,339 and Counting" in *Reports from the Holocaust*, p. 70.
55. Ibid., p. 73.
56. "The Scourge of a New Disease," *The New York Times*, May 15, 1983.
57. Henig, "AIDS: A New Disease's Deadly Odyssey."
58. Glenn Collins, "Facing the Emotional Anguish of AIDS," *The New York Times*, May 30, 1983, p. 14.
59. Kramer, *The Normal Heart*, p. 29.
60. Ibid., p. 96.
61. Collins, "Facing the Emotional Anguish of AIDS."
62. Dudley Clendinen, "AIDS Spreads Pain and Fear among Ill and Healthy Alike," *The New York Times,* June 17, 1983, p. A1.
63. Claudine Herzlich and Janine Pierret, *Illness and Self in Society*, trans. Elborg Forster (Baltimore and London: The John Hopkins University Press, 1987), p. 28.
64. Cindy Patton, "The New Right" in *While the World Sleeps*, p. 29.
65. Altman, "New Homosexual Disorder."
66. Michael S. Gottlieb, moderator, "The Acquired Immunodeficiency Syndrome," *Annals of Internal Medicine*, 99 (1983): 208–220, 217.
67. Kramer, "1,112 and Counting," p. 48.
68. Lockman, p. 48.
69. Kramer, "1,112 and Counting," p. 48.
70. Herman, "A Disease's Spread Provokes Anxiety."
71. Susan Sontag, *Illness as Metaphor and AIDS and Its Metaphors* (New York: Picador, Farrar, Straus and Giroux, 1989), p. 134.
72. Seligmann et al., "The AIDS Epidemic: The Search for a Cure."
73. Ibid.
74. Henig, "AIDS: A New Disease's Deadly Odyssey."
75. Lawrence K. Altman, "Five States Report Disorders in Haitians' Immune Systems," *The New York Times*, July 9, 1982, p. D15.
76. Lawrence K. Altman, "Debate Grows on US Listing of Haitians in AIDS Category," *The New York Times*, July 31, 1983, p. 1.
77. *MMWR*, November 30, 1984, 133(47): 661–664 and "The New Plague in Perspective," *The New York Times*, September 3, 1985, p. A20.
78. "Now No One Is Safe from AIDS," *Life*, 8, no. 8, July 1985, pp. 12–18.
79. "The New Plague in Perspective," *The New York Times*, September 3, 1985.
80. Ibid.

81. Sontag, p. 132.
82. *An Early Frost.*
83. Ibid.
84. "San Francisco Seeks to Combat Fear of AIDS," *The New York Times*, May 22, 1983, p. NJ1.
85. Ibid.
86. Arthur Reinstein, "Hysteria Is behind the Drive to Bar AIDS Victims from Schools," *The New York Times*, December 15, 1985, p. NJ40.
87. Shelly Feuer Domash, "AIDS Fears Cut Blood Donations," *The New York Times*, December 29, 1985, p. LI1.
88. Herzlich and Pierret, p. 46.
89. Perri Klass, "Hers," *The New York Times*, October 25, 1984, p. C2.
90. Ibid.
91. Ibid.
92. James Cross Giblin, *When Plague Strikes: The Black Death, Smallpox, and AIDS* (New York: Harper Collins Publishers, 1995), pp. 165, 166.
93. Lisa A. McGowan, "Haiti," *Foreign Policy in Focus*, January 1, 1997, http://www.fpif.org/reports/haiti.
94. Henig, "AIDS: A New Disease's Deadly Odyssey."
95. Altman, "Debate Grows on US Listing of Haitians in AIDS Category."
96. Ibid.
97. *MMWR*, May 10, 1985, 34(18): 245–248.
98. Henig, "AIDS: A New Disease's Deadly Odyssey."
99. Clendinen, "AIDS Spreads Pain and Fear among Ill and Healthy Alike."
100. Ibid.
101. Kramer, *The Normal Heart*, p. 100.
102. William Greer, "Violence against Homosexuals Rising, Groups Seeking Wider Protection Say," *The New York Times*, November 23, 1986, p. 36.
103. Ibid.
104. *MMWR*, September 20, 1985, 34(37): 561–563.
105. Andrew Holleran, "Friends at Evening" in *Vital Signs: Essential AIDS Fiction*, ed. Richard Canning (New York: Carroll and Graf Publishers, 2007), p. 8.
106. Kramer, "1,112 and Counting," p. 33.
107. Ibid., p. 50.
108. *An Early Frost.*
109. John A. Dorsey, "AIDS: Reason Clouded by a Plague Mentality," *The New York Times*, April 27, 1986, p. NJ28.
110. Ibid.
111. Ibid.

Chapter 7

1. C. Everett Koop, *Surgeon General's Report on Acquired Immune Deficiency Syndrome*, October 22, 1986, http://profiles.nlm.nih.gov/ps/access/NNBBVN.pdf.

2. Koop, p. 5.
3. Ibid.
4. Ibid., p. 23.
5. Ibid., p. 6.
6. Stephen J. Gould, "The Terrifying Normalcy of AIDS," *The New York Times*, April 19, 1987, p. SM32.
7. Koop, p. 12.
8. Burton Levine, "Connecticut Opinion; AIDS and Plague: False Comparison," *The New York Times*, May 31, 1987.
9. Edmund White, "An Oracle" in *Vital Signs: Essential AIDS Fiction*, ed. Richard Canning (New York: Carroll and Graf Publishers, 2007), p. 56.
10. "AIDS May Dwarf the Plague," *The New York Times*, January 30, 1987, p. A24.
11. James Kinsella, *Covering the Plague: AIDS and the American Media* (New Brunswick and London: Rutgers University Press, 1989), p. 102.
12. Robert Gallo, "The AIDS Virus," *Scientific American*, 256, no. 1 (1987): 47–56, esp. 47.
13. Ibid.
14. Robert C. Gallo and Luc Montagnier, "AIDS in 1988," *Scientific American*, 259, no. 4 (1988): 41–48, esp. 47.
15. A.M. Rosenthal, "Individual Ethics and the Plague," *The New York Times*, May 28, 1987, p. A23.
16. For these statistics see Randy Shilts, *And the Band Played On: Politics, People, and the AIDS Epidemic* (New York: Penguin Books, 1987), p. 596 and Allen White, "Reagan's AIDS Legacy: Silence Equals Death," *San Francisco Chronicle*, June 8, 2004.
17. Shilts, pp. 595–596.
18. Peter Goldman, "One Year in the Epidemic: the Face of AIDS," *Newsweek*, August 10, 1987, p. 22.
19. Ibid.
20. Ibid.
21. Gilbert Meilaender, *Morality in Plague Time: AIDS in Theological Perspective* (St. Louis: Concordia Publishing House, 1989), p. 14.
22. Ibid., p. 15.
23. Ibid., pp. 15, 16.
24. White, "Reagan's AIDS Legacy."
25. Shilts, p. 311.
26. *MMWR*, December 12, 1986, 35(49): 757–760, 765–766.
27. "AIDS Alarms, and False Alarms" *The New York Times*, February 4, 1987, p. A26.
28. Jon Nordheimer, "AIDS Specter for Women; The Bisexual Man," *The New York Times*, April 13, 1987, p. A1.
29. Bruce Lambert, "Unlikely AIDS Sufferer's Message: Even You Can Get It," *The New York Times*, March 11, 1989, p. 29.
30. Nordheimer, "AIDS Specter for Women."

31. Andrew Holleran, "The Absence of Anger" in *While the World Sleeps: Writing from the First Twenty Years of the Global AIDS Plague*, ed. Chris Bull (New York: Thunder's Mouth Press, 2003), pp. 102, 103.

32. Paul Monette, *Borrowed Time: An AIDS Memoir* (New York: Avon Books, 1988), pp. 18, 32.

33. Shilts, p. 147.

34. Ibid., p. 439.

35. Ibid., p. 113.

36. Kinsella, p. 159.

37. Shilts, p. 138.

38. Ibid., p. 165.

39. Richard Canning, introduction to *Vital Signs: Essential AIDS Fiction* (New York: Carroll and Graf Publishers, 2007), p. xxx.

40. Shilts, p. xxii.

41. Ibid., pp. xxi–xxii.

42. Ibid., p. 2.

43. Ibid., p. 596.

44. Ibid., p. 601.

45. Larry Kramer, "The Plague Years" in *Reports from the Holocaust* (New York: St. Martin's Press, 1989), p. 150.

46. Ibid., p. 158.

47. Larry Kramer, "I Can't Believe You Want to Die" in *Reports from the Holocaust*, p. 173.

48. Ibid., p. 163.

49. Larry Kramer, "The Beginning of ACTing Up" in *Reports from the Holocaust*, pp. 127, 128.

50. Ibid., p. 138.

51. A description of the **Silence=Death** movement can be found in the *Encyclopedia of AIDS* @ http://www.backspace.com/notes/2003/04/07/x.html.

52. Koop, p. 30.

53. Monette, p. 82.

54. Shilts, p. 377.

55. Carol Pogash, *As Real As It Gets: The Life of a Hospital at the Center of the AIDS Epidemic* (New York: A Plume Book, 1994), p. 200.

56. See Michael Kimmelman, "Bitter Harvest: AIDS and the Arts," *The New York Times*, March 19, 1989 for labeling AIDS activist art "agitprop."

57. See Nicholas Nixon and Bebe Nixon, *People with AIDS* (Boston: David R. Godine Publisher, 1991), pp. 14, 19–21.

58. See Robert Mapplethorpe's 1988 *Self-Portrait* @ http://www.mapplethorpe.org/porfolios/self-portraits.

59. Shilts, p. 12.

60. Sharon L. Bass, "Funeral Homes Accused of Bias on AIDS," *The New York Times*, November 15, 1987, p. CN1.

61. Monette, p. 113.

62. Pogash, p. 97.
63. Ibid., p. 129.
64. Ibid., p. 127.
65. Gallo, "The AIDS Virus," p. 56.
66. Goldman, p. 23.
67. Steven V. Roberts, "Reagan Approves Special AIDS Panel," *The New York Times*, May 5, 1987, p. A31.
68. Susan Sontag, *Illness as Metaphor and AIDS and Its Metaphors* (New York: Picador, Farrar, Straus and Giroux, 1989), pp. 121–122.
69. Monette, p. 149.
70. Peter Lewis Allen, "The Birth of the Helms Amendment: How a Single Pamphlet Started an AIDS War" @ http://writ.news.findlaw.com/commentary/200925_allen.html.
71. Anushka Asthana and Sam Rogers, "America to Remove HIV Visa Ban after Briton's Protest," *The Observer*, July 5, 2009.
72. See "US HIV travel ban lifted as Bush signs new AIDS bill," *Pink News*, July 31, 2008, and Jessica Green, "US HIV travel ban lifted today," *Pink News*, January 4, 2010.
73. "Science and the Citizen," *Scientific American*, 256, no. 1 (1987): 58–59, p. 58.
74. Tamar Lewin, "Rights of Citizens and Society Raise Legal Muddle on AIDS," *The New York Times*, October 14, 1987.
75. Ibid.
76. "Family in AIDS Case Quits Florida Town after House Burns," *The New York Times*, August 30, 1987.
77. Linda Saslow, "AIDS on the Job: Businesses Fight Fears and Prejudices," *The New York Times*, January 8, 1989.
78. Ibid.

Chapter 8

1. David Bret, "The Freddie Mercury Story: Living on the Edge" from Queens Archives: Freddie Mercury, Brian May, Roger Taylor, John Deacon, Interviews, Articles, Reviews @ http://www.queenarchives.com/index.php?title= Freddie_Mercury.
2. Even in 2008, a nurse working in a Florida clinic for AIDS patients and a doctor working in a clinic in Pennsylvania admitted they must be "selective" when referring patients to other doctors for procedures because many still are reluctant to treat them or simply will not. See Joe Darrah, "Surviving the Stigma: Despite advances in healthcare and education, those with HIV/AIDS often experience discrimination," *Advance for Nurses*, 8, no. 1, January 1, 2008, p. 29.
3. "HIV Prevalence Estimates and AIDS Case Projections for the United States: Report Based upon a Workshop—Appendix B," *MMWR*, November 30, 1990, 39(RR-16): 27–31 and "HIV Prevalence Estimates and AIDS Case Projections for the US: Report Based upon a Workshop—Appendix A," *MMWR*, November 30, 1990, 39(RR-16): 19–26.

4. "Appendix B," *MMWR*, November 30, 1990, 39(RR-16): 27–31.
5. Gina Corea, *The Story of Women and AIDS: The Invisible Epidemic* (New York: Harper Perennial, 1992), p. 17.
6. "Revision of the CDC Surveillance Case Definition for Acquired Immunodeficiency Syndrome," *MMWR*, August 14, 1987, 36(No. 1S).
7. "1993 Revised Classification System for HIV Infection and Expanded Surveillance Case Definition for AIDS among Adolescents and Adults," *MMWR*, December 18, 1992, 41(RR-17).
8. Philip Brian Harper, "Eloquence and Epitaph: Black Nationalism and the Homophobic Impulse in Responses to the Death of Max Robinson" in *While the World Sleeps: Writings from the First Twenty Years of the Global AIDS Plague*, ed. Chris Bull (New York: Thunder's Mouth Press, 2003), p. 221.
9. E.R. Shipp and Mireya Navarro's "Reluctantly, Black Churches Confront AIDS," *The New York Times*, 18 November 1991 and Appendix B," *MMWR*, November 30, 1990, 39(RR-16): 27–31.
10. Eric Eckholm, "Facts of Life; More than Inspiration Is Needed to Fight AIDS," *The New York Times,* November 17, 1991.
11. Corea, p. 220.
12. Ibid., p. 268.
13. Bruce Lambert, "Black Clergy Set to Preach about AIDS," *The New York Times*, June 10, 1989.
14. Lindsey Gruson, "Black Politicians Discover AIDS Issue," *The New York Times*, March 9, 1992.
15. Corea, pp. 4–5.
16. Gruson, "Black Politicians."
17. Harper, p. 237.
18. Michael Kelly, "A Delicate Balance: Issues—AIDS; AIDS Speech Brings Hush to Crowd," *The New York Times*, August 20, 1992.
19. Frank Rich, "Journal; Mary Fisher Now," *The New York Times*, May 4, 1995.
20. Jamie L. Feldman, *Plague Doctors: Responding to the AIDS Epidemic in France and America* (Westport, Connecticut and London: Bergin and Garvey, 1995), p. 56.
21. Ibid., p. 238.
22. Larry Kramer, "A 'Manhattan Project' for AIDS" in *While the World Sleeps*, p. 162.
23. Felicia R. Lee's "Making Days Live in Face of Death; At AIDS Residence, a Nurse Helps Poor, Drug-Addicted Patients," *The New York Times*, January 2, 1995.
24. Ibid.
25. Diane Ketchum, "About Long Island; Confronting a Great Tragedy, and Losing All Your Friends, *The New York Times*, August 29, 1993.
26. Peter Steinfels, "Catholic Orders Need 'Dramatic' Change to Survive, Study Says," *The New York Times*, September 20, 1992.
27. Tony Kushner, *Angels in America: A Gay Fantasia on National Themes* (New York: Theatre Communications Group, 1995), pp. 92, 93.

28. Douglas Crimp and Adam Rolston, "Stop the Church" in *While the World Sleeps*, p. 172.
29. Stuart Elliott, "The Nation; Madison Avenue Finds Courage to Ask: Want a Condom?," *The New York Times*, January 9, 1994.
30. E.R. Shipp and Mireya Navarro, "Reluctantly, Black Churches Confront AIDS," *The New York Times*, November 18, 1991.
31. Ibid.
32. Vincent Canby, "Manhattan's Privileged and the Plague of AIDS," *The New York Times*, May 11, 1990.
33. *Longtime Companion*, dir. Norman René, MGM, 1990.
34. Kushner, p. 93.
35. *Philadelphia*, dir. Jonathan Demme, Sony Pictures, 1993.
36. Ibid.
37. Corea, p. 48.
38. Ibid., p. 100.
39. Lamar Graham, "The Heretic," *GQ*, 63, no. 11, November 1993, p. 245.
40. Ibid.
41. Ibid., p. 246.
42. *Kids*, dir. Larry Clark, Lions Gate Studios, 1994.
43. Ibid.
44. Ibid.
45. Kushner, p. 49.
46. Ibid., p. 52.
47. Larry Kramer, *The Destiny of Me* in *Two Plays: The Normal Heart and the Destiny of Me* (New York: Grove Press, 2000), p. 135.
48. *Silence=Death*, dir. Rosa von Praunheim with Phil Zwickler, First Run Features, 1990.
49. Ibid.
50. Ibid.
51. Ibid.
52. Abraham Verghese, "Lilacs" in *Vital Signs: Essential AIDS Fiction*, ed. Richard Canning (New York: Carroll and Graf Publishers, 2007), p. 149.
53. Jane Gross, "Second Wave of AIDS Feared by Officials in San Francisco," *The New York Times*, December 11, 1993.
54. Ibid.
55. David Leavitt, "Gravity" in *Vital Signs*, p. 104.
56. Ibid., p. 106.
57. *Philadelphia*.
58. *And the Band Played On*, dir. Roger Spottiswoode, HBO, 1993.
59. See *MMWR*, November 19, 1993, 42(45): 869–872 for American AIDS statistics and see "Sixty percent increase in estimated AIDS cases worldwide; maintaining concern for epidemic in Asia," WHO, United Nations, November 1, 1995 @ http://www.hartford-hwp.com/archives/28/035.html for global statistics.
60. *Silence=Death*.

61. Abraham Verghese, "My Own Country" in *While the World Sleeps*, p. 280.
62. Kushner, p. 192.
63. Feldman, p. 58.
64. Nicholas Wade, "Method and Madness; the Next Plague, and the Next," *The New York Times*, September 25, 1994.
65. Bruce Lambert, "In Texas, AIDS Struggle Is also Matter of Money," *The New York Times*, January 5, 1990.
66. *Philadelphia*.
67. Ibid.
68. Lambert, "In Texas, AIDS Struggle."
69. Iris De La Cruz, "Sex, Drugs, Rock-N-Roll, and AIDS" in *While the World Sleeps*, p. 191.
70. Ibid., p. 192.
71. Diane Ketcham, "About Long Island; Confronting a Great Tragedy, and Losing All Your Friends," *The New York Times*, August 29, 1993.

Chapter 9

1. Albert Camus, *The Plague*, trans. Stuart Gilbert (New York: Vintage International, 1948), p. 116.
2. Susan B. Chambré, *Fighting for Our Lives: New York's AIDS Community and the Politics of Disease* (New Brunswick, New Jersey, and London: Rutgers University Press, 2006), p. 178.
3. Elyse Tanouye, "Pharmaceutical Consortium to Begin Clinical Trials of Combined AIDS Drugs," *The Wall Street Journal*, April 14, 1994, p. B8.
4. Michael Waldholz, "For First Time, Drug 'Cocktail' Seems to Eliminate HIV in Its Hiding Places," *The Wall Street Journal*, November 7, 1996, p. B8.
5. Andrew Sullivan, "Fighting the Death Sentence," *The New York Times*, November 21, 1995.
6. Andrew Jacobs, "The Diagnosis: H.I.V.-Positive," *The New York Times*, February 2, 1997.
7. See Gina Kolata, "New Studies Offer Powerful and Puzzling Evidence on Immunity to AIDS," *The New York Times*, September 27, 1996 and "Seeking Reasons for Disease Genes," *The New York Times*, December 3, 1996.
8. Kolata., "New Studies Offer."
9. J. Claiborne Stephens et al., "Dating the Origin of the *CCR5-Δ32* AIDS-Resistance Allele by the Coalescence of Haplotypes," *American Journal of Human Genetics*, 62 (1998): 1507–1515.
10. Camus, p. 272.
11. Adam Klein, "Keloid" in *Vital Signs: Essential AIDS Fiction*, ed. Richard Canning (New York: Carroll and Graf Publishers, 2007), p. 250.
12. Ibid., p. 245.
13. Ibid., p. 252.

14. See Jonathan Larson, *Rent: The Complete Book and Lyrics of the Broadway Musical* (New York: Applause Theatre and Cinema Books, 1996).
15. Ibid., p. 58.
16. Ibid., p. 17.
17. Ibid., p. 43.
18. Ibid., p. 14.
19. Ibid., p. 38.
20. Ibid., p. 69.
21. Ibid., p. 79.
22. Michael Cunningham, *The Hours* (New York: Farrar, Straus, and Giroux, 1998), p. 63.
23. Ibid., p. 131.
24. Ibid., p. 198.
25. Ibid., p. 16.
26. John Kelly, *Three on the Edge: The Stories of Ordinary American Families in Search of a Medical Miracle* (New York, Toronto, London: Bantam Books, 1999), p. 31.
27. "Robert Farber, 47; Known for AIDS Art," *The New York Times*, December 30, 1995.
28. Tony Kushner, *Angels in America: A Gay Fantasia on National Themes* (New York: Theatre Communications Group, 1995), p. 280.
29. "Entertainer, Denied Job Because He Has H.I.V., Settles Case," *The New York Times,* December 19, 1996, p. A15.
30. Andrew Sullivan, "When Plagues End," *The New York Times,* November 10, 1996.
31. Ibid.
32. Jacobs, "The Diagnosis: H.I.V.-Positive."
33. Peter Lewis Allen, *The Wages of Sin: Sex and Disease, Past and Present* (Chicago and London: The University of Chicago Press, 2000), p. 154.
34. "The Changing Face of AIDS," *The New York Times*, November 4, 1996, p. A26.
35. James Cross Giblin, *When Plague Strikes: The Black Death, Smallpox, AIDS* (New York: HarperCollins Publishers, 1995), p, 187
36. Michael B.A. Oldstone, *Viruses, Plagues, and History* (Oxford: Oxford University Press, 1998), p. 140.
37. Ibid., p. 142.
38. Ibid., p. 143.
39. Paul W. Ewald, *Plague Time: How Stealth Infections Cause Cancers, Heart Disease, and Other Deadly Ailments* (New York and London: The Free Press, 2000), p. 128.
40. Gina Kolata, "Scientists See a Mysterious Similarity in a Pair of Deadly Plagues," *The New York Times*, May 26, 1998.
41. "The Global Plague of AIDS," *The New York Times*, April 23, 2000.
42. Kary B. Mullis, Foreword to Peter Duesberg, *Inventing the AIDS Virus* (Washington, D.C.: Regnery Publishing, Inc., 1996), p. xiii.
43. Ibid., p. xii.

44. Robert C. Gallo and Luc Montagnier, "AIDS in 1988," *Scientific American*, 259, no. 4 (1988): 44.
45. Mullis, p. xiv.
46. Peter Duesberg, *Inventing the AIDS Virus* (Washington, D.C.: Regnery Publishing, Inc., 1996), pp. 175–195.
47. Ibid., p. 209.
48. *MMWR*, November 24, 1995, 44(46): 849–853.
49. Ibid.
50. Duesberg, p. 410.
51. Ibid., p. 411.
52. Ibid., p. 178.
53. Edward Hooper, *The River: A Journey to the Source of HIV and AIDS* (Boston, New York, London: Little Brown and Company, 1999), p. 169.
54. See Ewald, pp. 128–129.
55. Hooper, p. 252.
56. Hooper, p. 780.
57. Hooper, p. 189.
58. Hooper, p. 810.
59. Jeannette Farrell, *Invisible Enemies: Stories of Infectious Diseases* (New York: Farrar, Strauss, and Giroux, 1998), pp. 205–206.
60. Thomas Glave, "The Final Inning" in *Vital Signs*, p. 282.
61. Ibid.
62. Ibid.
63. Ibid., pp. 277–278.
64. Ibid., p. 278.
65. Ibid., p. 292.
66. Ainsley Maloney, "Taking it to the Streets: An HIV program in Delaware discovered a number of patients weren't accessing care, so it took care to them," *Advance for Nurses*, January 21, 2010 @ http://nursing.advanceweb.com/regional-articles/features/taking-it-to-the-streets.aspx?prg=2.

Chapter 10

1. Cathy J. Cohen, *The Boundaries of Blackness: AIDS and the Breakdown of Black Politics* (Chicago and London: The University of Chicago Press, 1999), p. xv.
2. Gil L. Robertson, Introduction to *Not in My Family: AIDS in the African-American Community* (Chicago: Agate, 2006), p. 1.
3. Bob Herbert, "A New Civil Right Movement," *The New York Times*, December 26, 2005.
4. Ibid.
5. Ibid.
6. Byron Cage, "Back to the Basics" in *Not in My Family*, p. 199.
7. Ibid., pp. 200–201.
8. *MMWR*, November 18, 2005, 54(45): 1149–1153.

9. Robi Reed, "Reality Check" in *Not in My Family*, p. 41.
10. Jacob Levenson, *The Secret Epidemic: The Story of AIDS and Black America* (New York: Pantheon Books, 2004), p. 8.
11. Ibid., p. 15.
12. Giovanni Koll and Jaime Gutierrez's "Stigma and Homophobia: Fueling the Fire," *The Body Pro: The Complete HIV/AIDS Resource*, Spring 2009 @ http://www.thebody.com/content/art54913.html.
13. J.L. King, *On the Down Low: A Journey into the Lives of "Straight" Black Men Who Sleep with Men* (New York: Harlem Moon, Broadway Books, 2004), p. 21.
14. Al Sharpton, "The Power of Truth" in *Not in My Family*, p. 46.
15. Cohen, p. 35.
16. Scott Jaschik, "A New HIV Alarm," *The New York Times*, January 16, 2005.
17. Sharpton, p. 45.
18. Ibid.
19. Cohen, p. 1.
20. King, p. 4.
21. Ibid., p. 114.
22. Phill Wilson, "The Way Forward" in *Not in My Family*, p. 69.
23. Elizabeth Simpson, "If You Are a Black Woman, Janet Hall Has Something to Tell You," *The Virginian Pilot*, June 24, 2007, p. 1.
24. *Life Support*, dir. Nelson George, HBO Films, 2007.
25. Robert Klitzman and Ronald Bayer, *Mortal Secrets: Truth and Lies in the Age of AIDS* (Baltimore and London: The Johns Hopkins University Press, 2003), p. 15.
26. Ibid., p. 52.
27. Ibid., p. 109.
28. Peter Applebome, "Dentist Dies of AIDS, Leaving Florida City Concerned but Calm," *The New York Times*, September 8, 1990.
29. Klitzman and Bayer, p. 110.
30. David J. Sterken, "Legal Advocacy: HIV-positive RNs Have Legal Rights and Must Protect Their—and Their Patients—Health," *Advance for Nurses*, November 20, 2006, p. 18.
31. Klitzman and Bayer, p. 111.
32. Susan Hunter, *AIDS in America* (New York: Palgrave MacMillan, 2006), p. x.
33. Anthony Lewis, "At Home Abroad; Bush and AIDS," *The New York Times*, February 3, 2001.
34. *MMWR*, December 1, 2000, 49(47): 1061.
35. "Persons below Poverty Level in the US, 1975–2007" @ http://www.infoplease.com/ipa/A0104525.html.
36. Bob Herbert, "In America; It Hasn't Gone Away," *The New York Times*, May 31, 2001.
37. Ibid.

38. Global population statistics are from the Department of Economic and Social Affairs Population Division, "World Population Monitoring 2001: Population, environment and development" (New York: United Nations, 2001), p. 1.

39. Hunter, p. xii.

40. Ibid., p. 201.

41. See Christine Gorman, "The Graying of AIDS," *Time*, August 14, 2006, p. 56.

42. Henry J. Kaiser Family Foundation Press Release, April 28, 2009. @ http://www. thebodypro.com/content/art51551.html.

43. See Hunter, pp. 1–14.

44. Ibid., p. 7

45. Ibid., p. 11.

46. Elisabeth Bumiller, "Under Pressure, Conservative Withdraws from AIDS Panel," *The New York Times,* January 24, 2003.

47. Ibid.

48. Matthew Mosk, "Schaefer Faults AIDS Patients: MD Official Defends Proposed Registry," *The Washington Post*, October 13, 2004, p. B1.

49. Klitzman and Bayer, p. 192.

50. Jen McCaffery, "Women Guilty of Not Disclosing HIV Status," *The Virginian Pilot*, June 10, 2010, p. 2.

51. Ibid.

Conclusions

1. The most current list of FDA-approved ARVs as well as those in development can be found. @ http://www.thebodypro.com/index/treat/antiretroviral_link.html.

2. "Expanded HIV Testing—Implementing the CDC Recommendations: Guidance for Nurses," *Medscape*, March 31, 2008 @ http://cme.medscape.com/viewprogram/9090_pnt.

3. Susan M. Chambre, *Fighting for Our Lives: New York's AIDS Community and the Politics of Disease* (New Brunswick, New Jersey, and London: Rutgers University Press, 2006), pp. 184–186.

4. "Expanded HIV Testing."

5. Ibid.

6. "CDC Wants HIV Tests for Everyone," CNN.com May 9, 2006 @ http://www. opposingdigits.com/forums/about1452.html.

7. David Brown, "AIDS Case in N.Y. May Not Be a Harbinger of Supervirus," *The Washington Post*, February 9, 2005, p. A9.

8. Anemona Hartocollis, "Final Mass for Last of the Catholic General Hospitals," *The New York Times*, May 1, 2010.

9. Anne Katz, "Gay and Lesbian Patients with Cancer," *Oncology Nursing Forum*, 36, no. 2, March 2009, p. 205.

Index